MAKING
THE MOST OF YOUR
VITAL ENERGY

# THE ART OF
# CHI KUNG

## WONG KIEW KIT

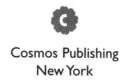

Cosmos Publishing
New York

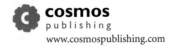

**cosmos** publishing
www.cosmospublishing.com

09 08 07 06 05 04    6 5 4 3 2 1

First published in United States and Canada in 2004 by Cosmos Publishing

Published in 1993 by Element Books
Published in 2001 by Vermilion

ISBN: 0-9749958-5-1

**Publisher's Cataloging-in-Publication**
(Provided by Quality Books, Inc.)

    Wong, Kiew Kit.
       The art of chi kung / by Wong Kiew Kit.
       p. cm.
       Includes bibliographical references and index.
       ISBN 0-9749958-5-1

      1. Qi gong.  2. Martial Arts.  3. Alternative medicine.  I. Title.

RA781.8.W66 2004         613.7'148
                 QBI04-200339

**DISCLAIMER:** While every care is taken to explain the techniques of Chi Kung clearly and systematically, neither the author nor the publisher can be held responsible for any injury or undesirable effects resulting from reading or practising the techniques mentioned in this book. Any attempt to apply them is the reader's own responsibility.
Nevertheless, you should not be unduly worried about this. Except for those advanced techniques where specific warnings are given, when treated with due respect practising Chi Kung is safer than walking down a road.

Cover Design by Michael Durkin – www.creativeoutlet.co.uk
Cover Calligraphy: Wong Kiew Kit
Distributed by Biblio Distribution

Printed in the United States of America on recycled paper

This book is dedicated to my beloved masters, Sifu Lai Chin Wah and Sifu Ho Fatt Nam, whose kind and generous teachings have made this book possible.

# CONTENTS

# PREFACE

Would you like to enjoy good health—physically, emotionally, mentally and spiritually? Would you like to increase your vitality so that you can get the best out of your work and play? Would you like to have clarity of thought and freshness of mind, as well as spiritual fulfillment? This book will show you, with examples and exercises, how you can attain all these goals—and more—with Chi Kung.

Chi Kung, as "qigong" is pronounced and traditionally spelt in English, is the esoteric art of energy training. This book will simplify the esoteric and make it comprehensible. It assumes no prior knowledge of Chi Kung: all terms and concepts are explained in a style and vocabulary that Western readers can readily understand. But you will be introduced, step by step, to all the important aspects of Chi Kung until, towards the end of the book, some fairly advanced concepts are introduced.

All the important dimensions of Chi Kung are discussed, namely:

1. The History, Philosophy and Scope of Chi Kung
2. Chi Kung for Health and Longevity
3. Vitality for Sports, Sex and Youthfulness
4. The Internal Force of Martial Arts
5. The Training of the Wonderful Mind
6. The Supreme Achievement of Chi Kung

As the scope of Chi Kung described in this book is extensive, you may select those sections that you find most appropriate or helpful, leaving others for later use or simply to read for pleasure. Because of cultural, philosophical and other differences, some readers may find certain descriptions unbelievable, even disagreeable. Suffice it to say that most of the examples mentioned in the book are verified by my students' and my own experience, and those that are outside our personal knowledge are quoted from great teachers and reliable authorities. Nevertheless I would ask you not to accept anything in this book on faith or reputation alone, but to approach the suggested principles and practices with an open mind, and to assess their benefits only after giving them a fair trial.

It must be emphasized that Chi Kung is essentially an experiential, not just an intellectual, discipline. It is not enough just to read and understand what Chi Kung is (though that itself is very beneficial); one must put in some practice if one is to appreciate and use the art fully. We need at least a few months of regular, consistent practice before we can even begin to play the piano competently—and a few months of practice before we could put on our clothes properly when we were young. It is therefore unrealistic and unreasonable to expect any proficiency in Chi Kung, or any art, if there is insufficient training.

Chi Kung is non-religious: it can be practiced by anyone without affecting their religious beliefs—or lack of them. At the more advanced levels it is spiritual—it transcends the physical—but there are many people who practice and benefit tremendously from its physical level only, leaving out some or all of the emotional, mental and spiritual aspects.

The exercises are introduced systematically but

it is unnecessary and inadvisable to practice all of them at once. Experience has shown that the best result is obtained by practicing only one technique—occasionally with one or two others to add variety, if you like—for at least a few months before proceeding to the next one.

While great care has been taken to explain the Chi Kung exercises in such a way that readers can learn from the book itself, it will be of great help if beginners can have an instructor's supervision. The instructor need not necessarily profess the same styles of Chi Kung as those mentioned in the book, as a sound knowledge of any style can provide the basic guidance. Those who cannot find an instructor will have to practice with more patience and prudence (but without undue hesitation or trepidation).

The ancient Chinese, like other great peoples of ancient civilizations, did not compartmentalize knowledge. Thus, many scientists and Chi Kung masters were also poets, and they often recorded their works in poetry. Many source materials quoted in this book were originally in poetic form, and the translations here are my own. If you do not find poetic beauty in these works, the fault lies in my translation, not in the original quality. In some instances, the original word order and syntax have been modified to facilitate rhyme and rhythm, but the original meanings have been maintained, as I believe that truth and beauty can, and often do, exist together.

One problem in writing this book—and possibly any other book where Chinese names are involved—is choosing a suitable method of transcribing names in Chinese characters into English spellings. The general principle I have adopted here is to use the official romanized Chinese spellings as far as possible, unless the English spellings have been universally accepted. Hence I use the romanized *Taijiquan* instead of the English spelling *Tai Chi Chuan*, but the English spelling "kungfu" instead of the romanized Chinese "gongfu" because although the term "Tai Chi Chuan" is known to many people, it is still not universally accepted, whereas "kungfu" is.

However my choice is sometimes arbitrary. For example, although my name is not universally known, I still prefer to use the English spelling, which is "Wong Kiew Kit," rather than the romanized Chinese, "Huang Qiao Jie," which I have to read twice before I can recognize it as mine.

This confusing difference is due to two factors. First, the English spelling of my name is based on Cantonese, my own dialect, which is used in South China and amongst overseas Chinese; whereas romanized Chinese is based on Mandarin, the official dialect which evolved from Pekingese and the Manchurian language. Secondly, the sound system of romanized Chinese is quite different from that of English. For example, "Qiao" is pronounced "Chiao," and "Jie" is pronounced "Jiet."

I have generally used terms like "man," "mankind" and "he," but they should be taken to mean "man and/or woman," "mankind and/ or womankind," and "he and/or she" respectively. I use such masculine terms simply to avoid the inevitable clumsiness of these latter expressions, and not through insensitivity.

It is my conviction that one of the best things I have ever done in my life is to practice Chi Kung. I hope you will share this conviction after reading this book. I have enjoyed every moment of writing and rewriting it, and I hope you will gain as much enjoyment, and derive as much benefit, as it is intended to provide.

Wong Kiew Kit
Grandmaster
Shaolin Wahnam Kungfu and
Chi Kung Institute

# FOREWORD

It is with great privilege that I write the foreword to *The Art of Chi Kung*. This is a book of excitement, joy, wonder, awe and hope, as it shares the ancient art of Chi Kung with us. For the total novice, this book reads simply and clearly and envelops one in the strength of the *chi*. We can barely read fast enough as this new world unfolds. For the master, this book complements already founded principles and techniques and clarifies what has remained hidden to so many.

*The Art of Chi Kung* is exemplified in the living example of Master Wong Kiew Kit. He bounces from an airplane, after a thirty plus hour flight, to present with a broad smile, glowing face and an alert and ready mind with no hint of jet lag. His world is always fresh and exciting. He leads by example and we owe him our gratitude as he so generously travels the world passing on this ancient art.

Please use this book as a guide and a map on your wondrous journey. Once we practice Chi Kung, we know we have found the excitement, joy, wonder, awe and hope for which we have been searching.

Jean Lie, R.N.
Toronto, Ontario
Canada

# PART ONE

# The History, Philosophy and Scope of Chi Kung

# CHAPTER ONE

# Exploring the Wonderful World of Chi Kung

The source of life, of birth and change is chi; everything under heaven and earth obeys this law. Chi in the periphery envelopes the cosmos; chi in the interior activates all.

*Nei Jing*

## Some Incredible Stories

"Come on, children," said Ratnam. "Let's go after the ball." They were actually his son's children, but nobody witnessing Ratnam's bouncing energy now would have guessed that only a year before this kindly grandfather had been suffering from a heart problem so serious that his specialist doctors wondered whether he would ever be able to walk again.

A pretty, young school teacher, Sharifah, knelt down and took a deep, slow breath. Then, in a flash, she smashed her hand on a brick. It broke— the brick of course, not the hand. There was loud applause. "How did she do it?" one of the surprised spectators commented. "She has such delicate-looking hands."

Talking to Chin, a senior government officer, could be frustrating or fascinating, depending on your attitude. He would often supply the answer to your question before you could ask it. "How do you do it?" he was often asked. "I read the question in your mind," he would reply with a smile.

These events occurred at different times, but they have one factor in common: the people concerned are my Chi Kung students, and they owe their energy or ability to the practice of this wonderful art.

## Uncovering Secrets

It is not surprising that many readers have never heard of Chi Kung. It is a very ancient art, but until the last twenty years it has been a jealously kept secret.

Chi Kung is written as "qigong" in romanized Chinese, with exactly the same pronunciation and meaning. But it would be a mistake to think that the romanized Chinese sound system is odd. Actually, the romanized Chinese spelling is more phonetically correct than the English spelling; the trouble lies in our unfamiliarity with it.

This diversion into phonetics illustrates a significant point: we often view with suspicion and disbelief whatever we are unaccustomed to, even though the unconventional may actually be better, and more acceptable, to other people. This observation is particularly pertinent as we examine the practice and philosophy of Chi Kung. It is therefore worthwhile for those who may not be used to the profundity of Eastern wisdom, and who may sometimes find it bewildering, to keep an open mind, and refrain from automatically dismissing as impossible or absurd patterns of thoughts and modes of behavior that are foreign to their culture.

### The Art of Developing Energy

Chi Kung is the art of developing energy, particularly for health, internal force, and mind training. In Chinese, energy is called *qi*, pronounced and often spelt as *chi* in English. *Chi* is the energy that enables you and me to walk and talk, to work and play, to philosophize and visualize, and to perform all the other myriad activities necessary for living. *Chi* is also the energy that changes the dinner you have just eaten into flesh and bones, that moves the necessary muscles when you smile, that fights the hostile microorganisms which invade your body, that transmits messages from your brain to various organs and tissues, and does countless other things inside your body that we are unaware of but that are essential to keep you and me and everyone else alive.

Of course, *chi* is not obtained from Chi Kung alone. People normally obtain their *chi*, or life energy, from the air they breathe and the food they eat. But practicing Chi Kung greatly enhances our energy, thus enabling us to get more out of life.

Besides keeping us alive—the most important function, and also the most easily forgotten—*chi* performs many other beneficial jobs too. There are three main areas, or dimensions, where Chi Kung is especially invaluable, namely: health, internal force, and mind training. For those who are ready, a fourth dimension may be added: spiritual fulfillment.

Chi Kung is excellent for curing illness and promoting health. There is a saying that Chi Kung can cure hundreds of illnesses. Understandably, many readers will consider this claim vain or exaggerated. The following chapters will not only explain why it is true, but also provide numerous case histories to support this apparently wild claim.

Internal force, obviously, is force from inside our body, and should be differentiated from external force, which is usually muscular or mechanical, and sometimes brutal. The young lady mentioned earlier, who could break a brick with her delicate hand, demonstrated an application of internal force. If you can work cheerfully and effectively from morning to evening, and yet still have energy to enjoy the night with your family, then you also exhibit internal force. Chi Kung develops internal force, and this book will show you how.

### The Training of Mind and Soul

The concept of mind-body unity has been prevalent in Eastern thought throughout the ages. Besides keeping the body physically fit and healthy, Chi Kung is preeminent in training the mind. The mental aspect in Chi Kung practice is important at all levels—though many beginners may not realize this—and it is greatly emphasized at the advanced stage, when fantastic feats can be achieved. The highly developed, intuitive mind of a Chi Kung master, probably more than any other single factor, is responsible for the many seemingly impossible feats that he can perform. Later in this book, you will find out how and why a master can perform what laymen would call miracles.

The supreme achievement of Chi Kung is spiritual fulfillment. Understandably, few people are ready for this stage; some may even consider such a development crazy! Whether or not you agree with this possibility, it is not my own theory or invention, but the crystallization of the thoughts and experiences of some of the greatest minds in history.

This supreme achievement enables you to actualize the innate immortality that has always been with you. You will achieve spiritual fulfillment, irrespective of what religion you profess, and even if you profess none at all. If you are a Christian, you will find the Kingdom of God; a Muslim, the return to Allah; a Hindu, union with Brahman; a Buddhist, Nirvana; a Taoist, unity with the Cosmos. Even if you claim that you do not believe in God, you will find yourself blissfully and spiritually merged into the Supreme Reality. If you are ready, you will intuitively understand and be joyously inspired by glimpses of such lofty experiences; if not, these words will merely sound hollow to you.

### Discoveries before History

Chi Kung is actually older than history. It was practiced in antiquity not only by the Chinese, but also by peoples of other great cultures at different places and times. It was known by different names. The Indians, for example, called it yoga; the ancient Greeks and Egyptians called it the art of mysteries; and the Tibetans, the art of wisdom.

The masters of these arcane, consecrated arts might not have heard of the term "Chi Kung," though all of them were quite similar in their aims, approaches, methodologies and philosophies. Like the Chinese, these ancient masters preserved their arts exclusively, teaching only a very few specially selected disciples. This explains why these arts developed independently.

Chinese archaeological records show that Neolithic cavemen in China practiced Chi Kung! Probably through trial and error, they discovered a number of Chi Kung techniques. For example, they discovered that if a person made an explosive sound at the point of m physical exertion, like saying "hert" when lifting a heavy object, he would be able to marshal more energy for the task; or if he gently exhaled on to an injured part of the body, like blowing "shssss" on to a wound, he would be able to relieve the pain.

### Imitating Animals and Internal Viewing

By the time of the Shang Dynasty (sixteenth to eleventh centuries BC), Chi Kung had developed to a fairly high level. Bronze vessels of this period show human figures in Chi Kung movements, which were perhaps the prototypes of today's Chi Kung patterns.

Many of the patterns of this time resembled the typical movements of animals, like the tortoise, the crane, and the monkey. Past masters believed that the characteristics of these animals, like the longevity of the tortoise, the steadiness of the crane, and the agility of the monkey, were related to the way they lived and acted. These and other physical movements that are meant to direct and lead internal energy flow are known as *dao yin*. So Chi Kung practitioners imitate the movements of animals not because they want to be bestial, but because they want to acquire particular characteristics which surpass those of humans.

The Zhou Dynasty (eleventh to third centuries BC) witnessed some very outstanding Chi Kung achievements. The famous *I Ching* (spelt as *Yi Jing* in romanized Chinese), or the *Book of Change*, introduced the concepts of *yin-yang* and *Bagua* (or *Pakua*), which later became essential elements in Chi Kung philosophy.

Those who are not familiar with the *I Ching* may think its divinations foolish or even ridiculous. But *I Ching* divination was often practiced by extremely powerful people, like generals and emperors, who were advised by some of the wisest men of the time.

Modern scientists and other great minds are beginning to realize that the *I Ching* is a book of profound wisdom, and that its copper-coin divination, like the augury of the Romans and the crystal-gazing of the Gypsies, is one way of triggering the subconscious to tap into the limitless resources of the Universal Mind.

The basis of *I Ching* divination is the *Bagua* (*Pakua*) or Eight Trigrams. The three lines of the *gua* or trigram are, of course, not just lines. Each *gua* is a physical symbol representing deeply metaphysical or subconscious manifestations. Every *gua* has a name, and the one known as *gen* represents man's various body parts and their functions.

It was meditating on this *gen* by Chinese sages that developed the supernormal skills of *nei guan* (internal viewing) or *nei jue* (internal reflection). These skills led to the growth of *cun xiang*, or thought retention, in Chi Kung. These three concepts are all generally translated as "visualization," but in Chinese there is a fine shade of difference between them. *Cun xiang* and *dao yin* evolved as the two principal directions of Chi Kung development.

### Opening the Way for the Gods

The Chinese language—a beautiful, poetic language to those who understand it—can present problems when Chi Kung terms are directly translated into English, an equally beautiful language in its own way.

Let us have a look at the sort of difficulty that can arise. There is a statement in the *Nei Jing* (*Inner Classic of Medicine*), which reads something like this when literally translated:

> Saints become attentive, eat air from the sky, and open the way for the gods.

It would be understandable if, based on such a translation, some readers considered the *Nei Jing* as something of a joke. But in Chinese medical circles the book is considered, even now, as one of the most authoritative texts on Chinese medicine. Such esteem becomes more meaningful when we understand the figurative meaning of the above statement as follows:

> The wise who know the arcane art go into deep meditation, breathe in cosmic energy, and through constant practice, eventually acquire supernormal abilities.

This arcane truth, which may still be difficult or vague to some readers, will become clearer in the course of this book.

The *Nei Jing* summarized the amazing achievements the early Chinese made in medical science prior to the Zhou Dynasty. It established a solid foundation for the philosophy and subsequent development of Chi Kung as well as Chinese medicine. Many of the principles mentioned in the *Nei Jing* can be very helpful to our modern doctors, if they care to study them a little more deeply. Let us take an example, one which lies at the very core of Chi Kung and Chinese medicine:

> Man is born of the chi of heaven and of earth, and is nurtured by the ways of the four seasons.

Although the translation is clear, many modern readers may still not understand the quotation. This is due to two factors: classical Chinese is concise; and words have deeper meanings than may superficially appear. The implication of the above quotation is as follows:

> The very substance of which a man is born is the same as the substance that comprises the whole universe—that is, energy. This energy may be manifested as different kinds, which are generalized into two main groups. The fine types are known as heaven energy, and the coarser types as earth energy.
>
> This energy, which is in man as well as in the whole universe, is not static. It is forever changing, and the changes can be brought about by different times and environments. The growth and development of a man, therefore, are affected by the seasons, which include not only climatic but also subtle psychological, physiological and other variations.

It must not be imagined that the above explanation is a matter of personal interpretation. All Chinese medical and Chi Kung students who have studied the *Nei Jing* will understand the quotation in this way, although the exact words may sometimes be slightly different.

The profundity of this concept, which is basic to Chinese medicine as well as to Chi Kung, becomes striking in comparison with modern conventional practice. For example, all patients suffering from a particular disease are generally prescribed the same medication by modern doctors, irrespective of whether they come from different physical and emotional environments or are undergoing different psychological and physiological changes. This philosophy of Western medicine, of diagnosing the *disease* and prescribing the appropriate treatment, contrasts sharply with the Chinese way, which is to treat the *patient* as a whole person and not just attend to the apparent disease.

Nevertheless, it is heartening to note that there is now a growing awareness amongst modern scientists of subtle cosmic influences on our lives. Lyall Watson, after providing much evidence from Western researchers, says:

> We wake and sleep, sweat and shiver, urinate and respirate in time with cosmic cues that are often so subtle that medical science has had a hard time taking them seriously. But an avalanche of studies during the last decade on insomnia, menstrual irregularity and stress in those suffering from cyclic disturbances such as jet lag, has turned the tide. It is now more widely accepted that functional integrity, the basic progresses of growth and control, and the efficient working of the central nervous system are all maintained to a very large extent by our electromagnetic environment.[1]

The profound Chinese concept of cosmic energy extends beyond medicine. It also explains why the Chinese, and many Eastern peoples in general, tend to follow rather than control Nature's ways. It is also the underlying principle explaining why

great Chi Kung masters, in special situations, can manipulate natural elements, and do things that seem inexplicable by natural laws. These and other fascinating topics will be discussed in more detail later in the book.

### Lifting The Sky for Health

Chi Kung is an experience, not just a gathering of knowledge. So practice is essential. The following exercise is one of the best in Chi Kung—beneficial to both the beginner and the master. Some variations in the technique, even some minor mistakes, are permissible. The form in Chi Kung is not an end in itself, but a means to induce energy flow inside the body. But it is of the utmost importance to breathe gently. A common mistake among beginners is to imagine that the more forcefully one breathes, the more powerful one becomes. That is not true. In Chi Kung training, what is breathed in is not just air, but cosmic energy, and forceful breathing often constricts the flow of cosmic energy. Another important point is to be relaxed. Keep your mind free from distracting thoughts while doing the exercise.

These three points are fundamental to all Chi Kung practice. But if you are a total beginner, even these may be difficult to follow. If that is so, don't worry. For the time being, just try to perform the exercise naturally.

Stand relaxed and upright with your feet fairly close together. Hold your arms straight down, with your hands at right angles to the forearm, and the fingers pointing towards each other, in front of you *(figure 1.1)*. Bring your arms in an arc forward and upward so that the palms, still at right angles, now face skyward *(figure 1.2)*. Breathe in gently through your nose as you do so. Look up at your hands. Gently hold your breath. Next, push your palms up, still at right angles, towards the sky. Then lower your arms sideways (*figure 1.3*), so that they return to your sides, gently breathing out through your mouth. At the same time lower your head to look forward.

Repeat this about ten to twenty times. Each time you push your palms to the sky, feel your back straightening. And each time you lower your arms, feel the flow of energy down your body.

This Chi Kung pattern is called *Lifting The Sky*. Like many other Chi Kung exercises, the form is deceptively simple, but what is significant is not the form itself, but the energy flow it induces. If you practice only this one exercise about ten times every morning without fail for three months, the results will be quite noticeable, and you will understand why it is one of the best in Chi Kung.

*Figs. 1.1–1.3 Lifting the Sky*

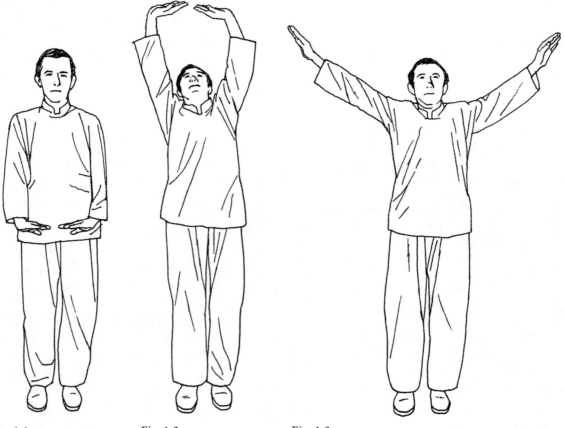

Fig. 1.1                    Fig. 1.2                    Fig. 1.3

# CHAPTER TWO

# Longevity, Poetry and Immortality

> The secret of immortality is to be found in purification of the heart, in meditation, in realization of the identity of the Self within and Brahman without. For immortality is union with God.
>
> *The Upanishads*

## What the Great Masters Said About Chi

Chi Kung is an ancient art and a modern science. Since earliest times, peoples of different cultures and locations have used cosmic energy for the purposes of promoting health, increasing vitality and developing the mind. This art of developing energy was most remarkable in great ancient civilizations like those of the Greeks, Egyptians, Indians and Chinese.

By the sixth century BC, the Chinese had successfully used Chi Kung in their search for health, longevity and immortality.

One of the greatest philosophers to have shown the way to immortality was Lao Tzu, the Patriarch of Taoism. One of his pieces of advice was: "Empty the heart, fill the abdomen." Some Western experts interpret this as meaning that if you fill the people's bellies, they will have no wish to revolt, which is reasonable. But actually, the saying is an arcane piece of advice on a fundamental Chi Kung technique:

Relax, and empty your mind and heart of all thoughts. Breathe in gently and deeply, so that the incoming cosmic energy fills the energy center at your abdomen.

We shall learn how to empty our hearts and fill our abdomens later in this book.

While Lao Tzu was esoteric, Confucius, the Patriarch of the Gentry, was more explicit. He advised:

A man of culture must observe three forms of abstinence. As a child, his chi [energy] has not been fully developed, so he must abstain from sex. As an adult, his chi is powerful, so he must abstain from aggression. As an aged person, his chi is weak, so he must abstain from greed.

Mencius, a philosopher regarded by Confucians as the Second Sage (Confucius being the First Sage), also provided invaluable exhortations on the practice and theory of Chi Kung:

The will is the commander of chi. Chi is the totality of the body.

Clear and direct though this statement maybe, it still needs some explanation in order for the layman to appreciate Mencius' remarkable insight. It may be expanded as follows:

Our willpower can control the flow of energy. When we think of a certain organ or area of our body, energy will flow to that part. Energy is the basic ingredient of our whole body. All our organs, tissues and cells as well as all our physiological functions and mental activities are the products of energy.

One cannot help marveling at how advanced the ancient Chinese were in their study and understanding of energy. These insights occurred two thousand years ago during the classical Zhou Dynasty.

### Would You Like to Gambol Like a Deer?

Numerous schools of thought on Chi Kung flourished during the Han Dynasty (third century BC to third century AD), but they could be classified into two major approaches which are still applicable today: the dynamic and the quiescent.

In Chinese medicine, Chi Kung became pre-eminent, emphasizing prevention rather than cure, although Chi Kung therapy was practiced with resounding success. Many of China's greatest doctors were also great Chi Kung masters. Hua Tuo, who is revered as the Saint of Chinese medicine, invented a set of Chi Kung exercises known as the *Five-Animal Play* with non-volitional movements (see *pages 35–36*) resembling those of the tiger, the deer, the bear, the monkey, and the bird.

Hua Tuo was a physician, a Chi Kung master, a physiotherapist and a surgeon. He successfully performed abdominal operations roughly 1000 years before Western surgeons even dreamt of such daunting feats. He taught the *Five-Animal Play* to his students who, though they were not sick, practiced the art diligently. The *Books of Later Han* recorded that not only were these students fit and healthy at ninety, but their eyesight and hearing were keen, and even their teeth, which still remained, were strong! If you want strong teeth when you are ninety, do not miss my explanation of *chi* flow exercises in Chapter 4.

Suppose you are suffering from an illness for which conventional Western medicine provides little help. As a last resort, you seek a Chi Kung therapist. He asks you to relax, which is an essential part of the procedure, and he opens some of your energy centers by gently touching certain points on your skin. Soon you start to move involuntarily. A little later, and apparently without having any say in the matter, you may roar like a tiger, dance like a monkey or gambol like a deer! You may even enjoy yourself while performing these antics, and after a few such sessions with your Chi Kung therapist, you could well find your chronic illness cured. This sounds incredible, but it is true.

### The Taoist Quest for Immortality

The type of Chi Kung developed by Hua Tuo and other great men of medicine can conveniently be termed the "medical school," and is effective for curing illness, improving health and promoting longevity. Taoist Chi Kung, on the other hand, transcends the physical, and aims at the development of mind and spirit. It teaches the unity of man's soul with the Universal Consciousness, thereby bringing immortality, and it attained great importance during the Han and post-Han periods.

If you do not agree with such concepts as Universal Consciousness and immortality, please ignore them and the relevant sections of this book. You can enjoy the physical, emotional and mental benefits of Chi Kung without modifying your personal beliefs. Nevertheless, the knowledge mentioned here is derived not from mere specu-lation, nor from philosophical reasoning, but from years of empirical studies and the experience of some of the greatest Chinese in history. And the Chinese people have been noted for their sense and pragmatism. You are invited to share this rare knowledge, but only if you want it. It is worth noting, however, that modern Western science has rediscovered many of the truths of Eastern wisdom. It is also important to note that terms like Taoist and Buddhist are philosophical, not religious, in significance. Chi Kung is strictly non-religious.

Taoist meditation, which is the essential paramount path to immortality, can be classified into two main methodologies, namely "one-pointed mind" and "visualization." The *Classic of Elixir* and the *Peace Classic*, two of the greatest Taoist Chi Kung texts of this period, gave elaborate accounts of these methodologies. The following extract from the *Peace Classic* illustrates a basic principle in Chi Kung as well as Taoist philosophy:

> We have a body, and this body is the unity of the physical and the spiritual. The form itself is dead; it is the spirit that gives the physical life. When there is normal harmony between the physical and the spiritual, it is propitious; if this harmony is disturbed, it is deleterious. If there is no physical substance, the spirit will wither; when there is substance, the spirit will flourish. Constant harmony unites the physical and the spirit into one. Constant illness causes the physical and the spirit to separate.

### The Real You before You Were Born

Buddhism spread from India to China during the Han Dynasty and Buddhist practice and philosophy greatly influenced and enriched Chi Kung.

A significant feature of Buddhist Chi Kung is its emphasis on mind training. Some Buddhist masters went so far as to say that our physical body is but "a smelly, skin-clad receptacle." Their aim, therefore, was to distill the mind, so that the real You—the You before you were born in this life—is liberated from its smelly prison.

Other Buddhist Chi Kung masters were less puritanical. Though they too regarded the mind as supreme, they also considered the physical body as important, at least while the real You is still living in it. So they first strengthened and purified the physical body, before they proceeded to purify the mind. One such great master was the Venerable Bodhidharma.

Like Gautama Buddha, Bodhidharma was also a prince who voluntarily renounced his worldly luxuries to lead, and help others lead, an even richer life. Bodhidharma came from India, and meditated for nine years at the famous Shaolin Monastery in China, founding Chan Buddhism, which later spread to Japan and the rest of the world as Zen Buddhism. Chan, or Zen, meditation became a very important aspect of Chi Kung.

Bodhidharma was also the first Patriarch of Shaolin kungfu, the famous martial art of China. Shaolin masters, as well as masters of other martial systems, used Chi Kung to enhance their fighting arts. This type of Chi Kung is generally known as the martial school, sometimes called *hard* Chi Kung. Some of the *hard* Chi Kung exercises you will find in this book were once taught at the world-renowned Shaolin Monastery.

### Chi Kung in Poetry and Medicine

The Tang Dynasty (seventh to tenth centuries AD) is best known for its poetry, and many poets were devoted Chi Kung practitioners. The great poet Po Chu Yi registered the sensations he experienced while in a meditative Chi Kung state:

> As I close my eyes to meditate
> Vibrant chi from within radiates.
> Tingling feelings of joy arise
> Like crawling insects in gentle surprise.
> This sensation permeates into every cell.
> From the center the void begins to swell.
> Forgetting myself and becoming formless,
> My mind and cosmos dissolve into nothingness.

Another great Tang poet, Tu Fu, described a Chi Kung mystic:

> He eats nothing but the cosmic juice.
> He thinks nothing except mist and smoke.
> Distinguished, illustrious, he prefers
> Living amongst wild ferns and mountain brooks.

While men of literature found *chi* a source of inspiration and truth, men of medicine regarded it as the very foundation of pathology—diagnosis as well as therapeutics. In AD 610, Chao Yuan Fang, the Imperial Professor of Medicine, edited the first specialist Chinese book on pathology, *Causes of Diseases*, in fifty volumes. This colossal work is also China's first specialist book on Chi Kung therapy. It recorded 1270 different kinds of illness, explaining the symptoms, causes and therapeutic principles of each. The extraordinary feature of this splendid work was that no appendices of herbs, drugs or other materia medica were included, as was the normal practice; instead about four hundred types of Chi Kung exercises were described as remedies for the various diseases!

Another authority on medicine at this time was Sun Si Miao, physician, scholar and Chi Kung master. By practicing Chi Kung, he lived over a hundred years, and wrote numerous theses on Chi Kung and medicine. He is well known for expounding the *Six Sounds* of Chi Kung therapy, which use different sounds affecting different organs to cure various diseases.

If you find this idea of sound therapy fascinating, *Chi Channeling* is equally so. Have you ever seen a therapist, in deep concentration, placing his palm motionlessly near his patient, or moving it as if stroking but not actually touching the patient's diseased area?

This is *Chi Channeling*—the therapist channeling his life energy into the patient to effect a cure. It is a very convenient and effective therapeutic method, and manifests a personal sacrifice on the part of the healer as he has to give away some of his life energy to the patient. The early Christian saints probably did the same thing when they performed miraculous cures. The great Franz Anton Mesmer, who was much misunderstood by his contemporaries channeled chi, which he called animal magnetism.

*Chi Channeling* as a therapeutic practice was very popular during the Tang Dynasty. The earliest existing thesis on it is *The Secret of Chi Channeling*, written in the eighth century AD by an unnamed author. The technique had been practiced in earlier periods, but because people did not understand its working then, it was often regarded with suspicion, and sometimes relegated to the realms of the supernatural. The book explained the principles and working of *Chi Channeling* in a rational way, thus restoring this useful therapy to a respectable position.

### Fantastic Skills and Wondrous Gateways

Chi Kung for martial arts became prominent during the Tang period. Shaolin kungfu, the most famous of the martial arts, recorded seventy-two specialized arts like *Golden Bell*, *Iron Palm*, and *Running on Grass-top*, which incorporated Chi Kung in their training. So, if you have ever wondered how a Shaolin master can take punches without suffering an jury, break bricks with his bare hands or run extremely fast and long without feeling tired, the secret is *chi*. Some of these fantastic skills will be discussed in some detail in Chapter 13.

During this period, Chinese Buddhism reached its full bloom. Buddhist meditation, which is aimed at achieving enlightenment, can also induce psychic or paranormal powers, like telepathy, clairvoyance, prediction and mind-projection. While Buddhist purists consider these powers a diversion in their quest for enlightenment, many

Chi Kung masters believe that they can be used benevolently to benefit humanity.

The highly reputed *Six Wondrous Gateways to Meditation*, more often heard of than understood, were formalized at this time by Zhi Yi. If you are interested in meditation but have difficulty in taming your mind, you will find the first two gateways extremely useful. However, if you want to advance, it is advisable to train under a qualified instructor.

The *Six Wondrous Gateways* are: Count, Follow, Tranquil, Watch, Repeat, Still. Briefly the method is as follows. Sit cross-legged, or comfortably upright, and relax. Close or half-close your eyes. *Count* your breathing in sets of ten. Then *follow* the inward and outward flow of your breath. Be *tranquil*. If you feel drowsy, *watch* your breaths in your mind's eye. If distracting thoughts enter your mind, *repeat* the whole process. Ultimately, attain wisdom in *stillness.*

Like many other Chi Kung techniques, the method appears simple. But if you can do it well over a period of years, you will achieve results that you would never have thought possible, even in your wildest dreams. The Buddha attained his enlightenment using this method.

## Secrets in the Clouds

If you wanted to study the most important Taoist Chi Kung texts prior to the Song Dynasty (tenth to thirteenth centuries AD) a good choice would be *Secrets in the Clouds*—if you understand classical Chinese. This rare collection of 120 volumes is an abridged version of *Precious Collections of the Great Song Heavenly Palace*, consisting of 4500 volumes—the colossal result of an imperial order to collect and edit all valuable Taoist texts prior to that period. Even in the shorter version, you would find almost any Chi Kung techniques you could imagine, including some interesting ones like

*Tortoise Technique, Absorbing the Moon's Essence,* and *Fetus-breathing Method.*

The *Precious Collections* was surpassed in the Ming Dynasty (fourteenth to seventeenth centuries AD) by the *Taoist Collections*, consisting of 5485 volumes. The *Grand Collections of Ancient and Modern Books and Pictures* and the *Great Encyclopedia of Everlasting Happiness*, which contained a tremendous amount of Chi Kung materials, were even more gigantic; they consisted of 10,000 and 22,817 volumes respectively! This gives a good idea of the advancement of Chi Kung and the enormous amount of literature recorded. But the common people, of course, had little access to this rich knowledge.

Great men of literature of the Song Dynasty, like Su Tung Po, Lu You and Au Yang Shiu, not only practiced Chi Kung diligently, but also recorded their experiences of, benefits from, and thoughts on Chi Kung in their poems and essays. If you are still young but feel old, or if you have reached three score years and ten, but still want to be young, these lines from Lu You's poetry will provide some hope and inspiration:

> Happiness is health and living without rush.
> At sixty I climb mountains without a crutch.
> Nearing ninety chi's made me fit and strong.
> With a thousand books my eyes still dance along.

## Carrying The Moon for Youthfulness

Obviously, merely reading the above poem, hopeful and inspiring though it may be, will not make you youthful. But regularly practicing the following Chi Kung exercise will, as has been proven by many students. It is called *Carrying The Moon.*

Practice the exercise in the open air if possible. Wear something loose and comfortable, so that your clothing will not hinder *chi* and blood

*Figs. 2.1–2.4 Carrying the Moon*

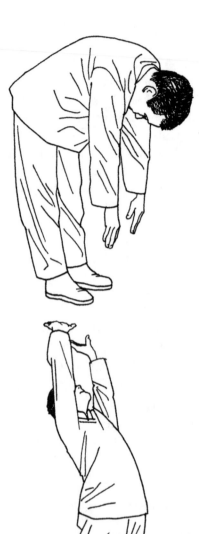

*Fig. 2.1*

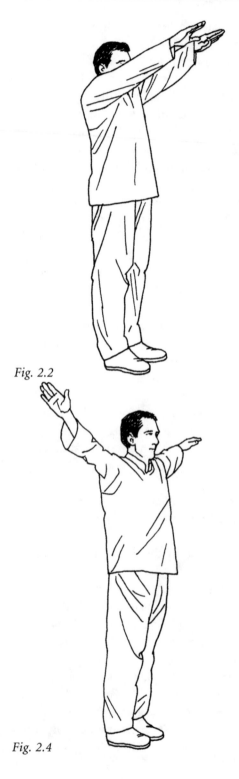

*Fig. 2.2*

*Fig. 2.3*

*Fig. 2.4*

circulation. These and the points mentioned in the previous chapter—relaxed, gentle breathing and a clear mind—apply to all Chi Kung exercises.

Stand upright but relaxed. Then bend your body forward so that your arms drop effortlessly in front, and your fingers are slightly below knee level, as in *figure 2.1*. Keep both arms and legs straight. Tuck your head in so that your back forms a continuous curve. Gently hold your breath. Think of your *chi* flowing from your anus up your spine to the crown of your head.

Then straighten your body slowly, lifting your arms, with the elbows straight (see *figure 2.2*), in a continuous arc to the front and then up above the head. Simultaneously breathe in gently through your nose. When your hands are above your head, bend your arms slightly, and form the shape of a full moon with both thumbs and index fingers.

Continue the body movement backwards so that your back bends in an arc with your hands forming the round shape of the moon beyond your head (see *figure 2.3*). Hold the pose, and your breath, for two or three seconds. Then straighten your body and lower your arms from both sides (see *figure 2.4*), simultaneously breathing out gently through your mouth. Visualize *chi* flowing from your head down your whole body like a cascade or waterfall to your fingertips and toes. Feel the pleasant, tingling sensation as it flows inside your body. Think of this waterfall of vital energy cleansing your body of rubbish (negative emotions, illness, toxic waste, and such like) own into the ground through your soles, and at the same time let the vital energy nourish every cell in your body, making you healthy and youthful. Remain motionless for a second or two to enjoy the pleasant sensation of energy flow. This completes the sequence. Repeat it about ten to twenty times.

*Carrying The Moon* may be performed on its own or in combination with other exercises. You may, for example, start with six sequences of *Lifting The Sky*, followed by six sequences of *Carrying The Moon*. As you progress, you may gradually increase the number of times you do the exercise, and be surprised that you are growing younger each day!

# CHAPTER THREE

# From Ancient Wisdom to Modern Science

There is one common flow, one common breathing. All things are in sympathy.

Hippocrates

### The Amazing Cosmos

Many people are surprised to discover how advanced the ancient Chinese were in their knowledge of the universe. Not only did they have amazing knowledge of the stars and their influence on human affairs, but they also had a profound understanding of the subatomic dimension. But how could they know about the subatomic world when the bubble-chamber in which the atom was broken down was not invented until the twentieth century? The past masters used mankind's finest instrument—the mind in deep meditation.

Through meditation, a Song Dynasty scientist, Shao Yong, worked out the theoretical structure of the universe. The following poem by him, reminiscent of William Blake who lived more than seven centuries later, captures the reality of *chi* in an intense moment of inspiration:

The universe is like our body,
    The cosmos in our hand.
Nebulous, formless they remain
    Manifested in forms without end.

Zhang Dai, another Song Dynasty scientist and Chi Kung philosopher, was more explicit. Modern physicists would be amazed at what this great man said almost a thousand years ago:

The cosmos is a body of chi. Chi has the properties of yin and yang. When chi is spread out, it permeates all thing; when it coalesces, it becomes nebulous. When this settles into form it becomes matter. When it disintegrates, it returns to its original state.

### The Golden Pearl of Energy

Many Chinese scientists were influenced by Taoist thought. Two great Taoist masters of this time were Wu Chong Xu and Liu Hua Yang, who successfully combined the best of Taoist and Buddhist meditation, and passed on to us a splendid methodology that is still much used today. The following is a summary of a once highly secretive technique taught to the Emperor in his quest for immortality. It is, of course, written in symbolic language, an effective way to

16

prevent such arcane knowledge leaking to the uninitiated. Have some fun trying to decipher it before reading the explanation below:

> The furnace must have a broad base and be erected upright. Mercury is infused as the main ingredient. The water that is added must come from a clean source. The fire that heats the ingredients must be of the right temperature. Lead, the waste product, is vaporized. The ingredients must be heated for three hundred days. If everything goes correctly, the ingredients will be purified into glittering real gold, which will be stored at the lower level of the furnace for further use.

Anyone not initiated into the secrets can easily misinterpret this as an alchemist's method for changing base metals into gold. Actually, it is a symbolic description of cosmic Chi Kung breathing for developing a pearl of energy. The real meaning is as follows. The furnace is the adept himself. He sits upright in a cross-legged position, so as to have a broad base. Mercury, being shiny, represents beneficial cosmic energy. Water represents intrinsic energy from the kidneys; a clean source means that the adept must be free from distracting thoughts during the Chi Kung training.

Fire represents intrinsic energy from the heart; the "right temperature" denotes that the breathing must be gentle. Chi Kung masters believe that intrinsic energy from the kidneys and the heart is required to produce the vital life force.

Lead, which is of a duller color, represents the unwanted energy in the body that is disposed of as waste products. The breathing practice, which circulates the cosmic energy round the body in a continuous flow known as the *Small Universe*, is maintained for 300 rounds. If the practice is done correctly, energy can be accumulated at the lower energy center at the abdomen. Here, the cosmic energy so developed, forms into a golden pearl radiating with life, and is ready for use in the subsequent training to achieve sainthood.

## The Art of Longevity

The Qing Dynasty and the Republics (from the seventeenth century onwards) mark the modern age of Chi Kung history. Many books on Chi Kung have been written in this period; most are for the prevention and cure of various diseases, some concern principles and philosophy and others deal with techniques and experiences. If you want a long life—and who doesn't?—the following method from Gong Ting Xian, in his *Achieving Longevity and Preserving Primordiality*, will be useful:

> Every time between 11 PM and 1 AM, 11 AM and 1 PM, 5 AM and 7 AM, and 5 PM and 7 PM, retreat to your meditation chamber. Place a warm mat on your wooden bed. Sit cross-legged and close your eyes. Use some cotton wool to block your ears. Do not have any thoughts. Be mindful of your breathing, following each inward and outward flow to a point between the heart and the kidneys. Do not be too fast, nor too slow; be natural. After sitting for the time of one incense,* you will find that your breathing through your mouth and nose has ceased to be rough, and has become smooth and gentle. After sitting for another incense, you will find no breath passing through your mouth and nose. Then gently stretch your limbs, open your eyes and take out the cotton wool. Leave your bed and walk about. Then lie on your wooden bed and take a nap. When you awake, eat half a bowl of light porridge. Do not work laboriously nor be angry, as this will diminish the effect you have acquired in the training. Practice the method every day. After two months, you will see the results.

## A Song for Lovemaking?

One important thinker of the early Qing period was Wang Fu Zhi, known to his scholar friends as Mr. Boat-Mountain. One of his outstanding

*That is, the time taken for one stick of incense to be burned, or about half an hour.

works is *Sixteen Songs of Dream Interpretation*, which is a commentary on the *Classic of Elixir*, the great masterpiece of Taoist Chi Kung. What do you think of one of these songs, entitled "Dragon Swallowing Tigress' Marrow?"

> Without a suitor the chaste lady remains alone.
> Even her chamber curtains and cold flowers moan.
> Like a fragrant duckling her figure pines away.
> At evening, pulses of inspiration congest and stay.
> Pushing and retreating she demurely entwines
> Into the lover's heart like white moonshine.
> Merging thoroughly like a mystical dream,
> The willow sways in spring breeze besides a stream.

If you think this is a romantic poem or a poem suggestive of lovemaking, you are in good company. But many others regard it as a serious description of an advanced technique in Chi Kung training. Unlike Chinese medical texts, which are both precise and concise, Taoist writings are deliberately concealed. I will leave the challenge of interpreting the poem for you to enjoy. It is likely that as you progress in the reading of this book, you will appreciate it at different levels of understanding.

### Chi Kung as an Umbrella Term

The term "Chi Kung" is actually a modern one. It was mentioned in the Han period, but its usage was not popular. It has become widely accepted only since the 1950s, when the great master Liu Gui Zhen published his influential book *Practical Chi Kung Therapy*. Since then the name has been extensively used as an umbrella term to cover all those arts that are concerned with *chi* or energy.

I have applied the term to all the earlier arts of energy, though at their time these arts were known by different names. Some of these names may sound strange or even ridiculous when translated literally into English, as is often the case

in English Chi Kung books. But in the original Chinese language, they are precise, and sometimes poetic. Here are some examples: *Eating Six Energies*, *Heel Breathing*, *Focusing One*, *Entering Silence*, *Tortoise Motion* and *Traveling Dragon*. Now let us look at their idiomatic beauty.

### The Different Names of Chi Kung

Ancient masters discovered that, because of the different positions of heavenly bodies and because of various factors on earth, there were six major types of energy in the universe and in man. *Eating Six Energies* is thus the art of developing these different energies.

*Heel Breathing* refers to a technique of deep breathing. Because of the comprehensive network of the body's meridians, energy breathed in through the nose can reach the heel, if we know how to do it. This technique was widely used by Confucian scholars.

"One" can mean the infinitesimally small or the infinitely big. *Focusing One* was a fundamental Taoist technique in their quest for immortality. Basically, it involves focusing the mind on the One, which can be an infinitesimal point inside oneself or the boundless indefinite cosmos. Confucian scholars also used this method to enhance their mental faculties.

"Silence" in *Entering Silence* refers to a subconscious level of mind attained in meditation. This method is usually practiced in a cross-legged or another comfortable sitting position. But the process of attaining silence, which is fundamental in all Chi Kung practice, can be carried out in any position, whether sitting, standing, lying down or even moving.

The tortoise has been noted for its longevity. Chi Kung masters believe that this is related to its mode of breathing. *Tortoise Breathing*, therefore, is a technique modeled on the tortoise's way of breathing, not on its appearance or the way it moves. So do not look down on any lowly creatures; they may teach us a thing or two.

The dragon is a divine, benevolent creature in Chinese culture. *Traveling Dragon* is a Chi Kung technique in which internal energy flow is induced by external movements, and the practitioner sways about gracefully and involuntarily, like the mystical dragon moving about in heaven. It is a very useful method for cleansing body toxins.

### The Material Reality of Chi

Despite the marvelous results of Chi Kung over the ages, many people have still been skeptical about *chi*, because it is not normally visible to the naked eye. Some regarded Chi Kung as superstitious, relegating its success to supernatural forces. Others thought that *chi* was a product of the imagination, alleging that cures were the happy consequence of psychological factors.

In 1977, researchers in China, using modern scientific apparatus, discovered that the *chi* transmitted by a Chi Kung master consists of electromagnetic waves, static electricity, infrared rays, and certain particle flows. It provided scientific evidence to establish, once and for all, what Chi Kung masters had claimed throughout the ages, namely that *chi* has a material reality.

So, if you are tempted to ask, "Where is chi? I cannot see it!" gently remind yourself that the fault actually lies in your eyes. Our eyes are very limited; they can only see an extremely narrow range of the light spectrum. X-rays, gamma rays, sound waves and radio waves, for example, are not visible to our eyes. We cannot even see the countless number of bacteria and viruses that are literally floating all around us.

### The Current Blossoming of Chi Kung

Chi Kung is going through a time of blossoming. Never before in history has there been a time when so many methods were introduced to the public, and so much Chi Kung information exposed. This blossoming was unthinkable in the past, when Chi Kung secrets were jealously guarded. It is quite amazing that nowadays an interested reader can go to a good bookshop and buy a Chi Kung text for which people in the past would have been ready to exchange their fortunes or risk their lives.

What caused the drastic change of attitude? One very significant factor is the philosophy of the government of the People's Republic of China, which stipulates that such things should not be kept exclusively for a select few, but must be shared by the common people.

The Chinese government set up special committees to study and spread Chi Kung at provincial and national levels. Following resounding successes in its use for curing illness, Chi Kung therapy is now widely used in hospitals. Instruments have been invented which can emit rays resembling the *chi* channeled by Chi Kung masters. In 1980 the Eighth People's Hospital in Shanghai successfully applied *chi*, and nothing else, as anesthesia in surgical operations!

Research scientists collaborating with Chi Kung experts have discovered many startling effects of practicing Chi Kung on physiological and psychological functions, validating the claims of past masters. For example, using modern scientific apparatus and methods, it has been found that practicing Chi Kung greatly enhances a person's natural defensive, regenerative and immune systems.

Some of the attainments of Chi Kung masters are incredible. For example, in December 1986, under scientifically controlled conditions at the prestigious Qing Hua University in Beijing, the great Chi Kung master Yan Xin demonstrated that he could transmit chi over 2000 kilometers to change the molecular structure of various liquids! The supernormal abilities of some Chi Kung masters were so fantastic that many uninformed people thought they were witches or saints.

Professor Qian Xue Sen, the father of the Chinese rocket, was so impressed with the achievements of Chi Kung that he suggested it as the key to the scientific study of man. He believed that this century's greatest breakthrough in medicine would be made through Chi Kung.

Since the 1970s, Chi Kung has become popular in many countries outside China. In Japan and Korea, both dynamic Chi Kung exercises and static meditative techniques are widely practiced. In Southeast Asian countries, dynamic exercises are more popular among the masses. In the USA and Europe, Chi Kung research centers have been established in numerous universities.

Some people have the misconception that Chi Kung is just some form of gentle physical exercise meant for maintaining health, and perhaps curing some diseases. This is a very limited view. Gentle physical exercise forms only a small part of Chi Kung. A similar situation occurred in yoga some years ago, when many Westerners thought of it as a series of funny postures meant for slimming or increasing sexual performance. While these benefits are true, they are very petty when compared to the wider aim of yoga, which is the union with God. In the same way, for one reason or another, many people only partially understand Chi Kung, not realizing the tremendous breadth and depth it can offer.

## The Very Essence of the Universe

In its widest sense, Chi Kung, as a study of *chi*, is concerned with all human activities that have anything to do with energy, including *feng shui* or geomancy, occult arts, spiritual sciences, phys-iognomy and climatology. In practical terms, however, Chi Kung is particularly concerned with maintaining health, enhancing martial arts, training mental faculties, and realizing spiritual fulfillment. The concern of Chi Kung is actually boundless, because *chi* is the very essence of the smallest subatomic particle, of man himself, and of the infinite universe.

Though they have developed independently, many disciplines of mind training, studies of psi and alternative healing systems have elements in common with Chi Kung. For example, the philosophy and methods used in Transcendental Meditation and Silva Mind Control are reminiscent of those of Chi Kung meditation. Telepathy, clairvoyance, psycho-kinesis and out-of-body experiences are phenomena that occur in Chi Kung too. Physiotherapy, chiropractic, reflexology, bio-feedback, Reiki, laying on of hands, faith healing, rebirthing and channeling use tech-niques that are also found in Chi Kung.

It is not surprising that Chi Kung is so extensive and comprehensive, because it is actually an umbrella term covering many arts dealing with energy. Hence, when you study and practice Chi Kung, you involve not only the very core of your being, but also the very essence of the universe.

## Relaxation—the First Step to Intuitive Wisdom

Long before modern science learned that matter and energy are actually two aspects of the same reality, Chi Kung masters in antiquity—and also great sages of other ancient cultures—already had knowledge of this timeless truth. The scientists arrived at truth by way of the intellect, with the help of precision instruments and gigantic observatories. The ancients had no exterior tools; they reached the same conclusion by way of intuitive wisdom using their own minds in deep levels of meditation.

Before you can meditate effectively, you must relax. Relaxation, therefore, is the first step to intuitive wisdom.

Even if you are not interested in intuitive wisdom, the ability to relax is in itself useful. First, if you can relax, you will be able to prevent, or even begin to reduce, many of the health and other problems troubling you. Secondly, relaxation will enhance your efficiency, improving both your work and your play—and even your sex life, if you want to add more color to it. Thirdly, relaxation is an essential element in Chi Kung practice. Most Chi Kung exercises, which bring tremendous benefits, are performed in a relaxed manner.

Relaxing is not difficult, if you know how, and the following method shows you.

Stand with your feet fairly close together in a peaceful, quiet place. Let your arms drop effortlessly at your sides. Close your eyes and eliminate all thoughts. Then follow the seven steps to relaxation:

1. Relax your head. Feel your face muscles and even your hair relax.
2. Relax your shoulders. Jerk them if you need to.
3. Relax your chest and the front part of your body. Feel how natural your breathing is.
4. Relax your back. Feel all the muscles loosen.
5. Relax your upper limbs right down to the finger tips. Wriggle your fingers if you wish.
6. Relax your lower limbs right down to your toes. Feel all your tension running out of the soles of your feet.
7. After you have relaxed your whole body, relax mentally. Feel that you do not have a care in the world, nor a thought in your mind.

These seven steps take only about two minutes to perform, but you can take your own time going through them. After you have relaxed physically and mentally, remain in this joyous, tranquil state of *Standing Meditation* (see *figure 3.1*) for about five minutes, or for as long as you feel comfortable. But do not continue for too long, or you may fall asleep!

Because I started training at an early age, relaxation has always come naturally to me. Hence, in the course of my teaching, I was very surprised to find that many adults had great difficulty relaxing. Nevertheless, all my students have been able to do it after learning Chi Kung from me. You too can share the bliss of relaxation if you follow this technique.

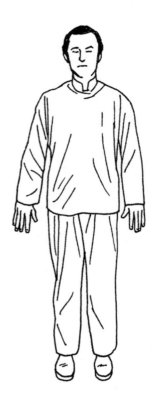

*Fig. 3.1 Standing Meditation*

# PART TWO

# Chi Kung for Health and Longevity

# CHAPTER FOUR

## "Incurable" Diseases Can Be Cured

> The idea of biological energy is developed to a greater or lesser degree in different therapies, but probably finds its most sophisticated expression in traditional Chinese medicine where this energy is termed chi....It comes as something of a surprise to realize that conventional medicine is the only medical system ever known to man which has no concept of biological energy.
>
> Dr. Julian N. Kenyon

### The Wonderful Flow of Chi

Lau, a young man of thirty, had a good job, no financial worries, and was unmarried. Yet he attempted suicide twice. Why? He was never jilted. He was not psychotic. He was not suffering from a terminal disease. But he was tormented by excruciating rheumatic pain for years.

He had seen many specialists, but all they gave him, to quote his own words, were "pills, pills and more pills." He had taken so many painkillers that they no longer had any effect on him. When the pain became unbearable, he literally banged his head against a wall. As a last resort, he tried Chi Kung therapy.

A Chi Kung master, Chan Chee Kong (who is what is known as my inner-chamber disciple, meaning a specially selected disciple), opened energy points on his body, and channeled *chi* to him. Chan also taught him Chi Kung exercises, including *Lifting The Sky* and *Carrying The Moon*, and induced the flow of *chi* in his body.

For the first month, there was no visible effect. Then Lau felt the *chi* moving in his body. Gradually the flow became so vigorous that he could hardly control his own movements. After four months, his rheumatic pain disappeared. He said to Chan Chee Kong, "How could I have been so silly as to think of committing suicide?"

Fantastic? No. In fact, the relief of rheumatism is a typical response to Chi Kung therapy, though Lau's was one of the more severe cases.

Let us look at another apparently fantastic case history. Steven, a schoolboy of fifteen, had suffered from asthma since early childhood. Though he lived in tropical Malaysia, he could never sleep with his windows open at night; he could not go out in the rain or drink cold water, otherwise, he would have an asthma attack. It appeared that his condition was hereditary. Again, he had consulted numerous specialists, but to no avail.

Chim Chin Sin (another of my inner-chamber disciples and a Chi Kung master) taught Steven some Chi Kung exercises. He also opened some energy points and induced the flow of energy. In the second week, pus flowed from Steven's eyes and toes. After another week, all his asthmatic symptoms disappeared. He has had no attacks since. His was one of the fastest recoveries in our records.

## Miracles Do Happen

Let us look at an even more amazing case—so amazing that very, very few people would believe it, although it really did happen.

Jane telephoned me from Australia. "Sifu," she said. "I'm going blind! Two eye specialists have confirmed it. One said I'd be blind in two weeks; the other gave me two months."

"What do they recommend?" I asked. Jane had returned home recently after learning Chi Kung from me in Malaysia to have her kidney cancer cured, which it was.

"They couldn't do anything. One of them suspected that the nerves serving my eyes are not functioning. He recommended me to go to the States for a brain scan. It's expensive and risky. The worst is the scan can't prevent my blindness; it will merely confirm what he suspects."

The first thing that troubled me was the thought that somehow her learning Chi Kung from me had contributed to her impending blindness, though I knew very well it could not have done. "Are you going for the scan?" I asked.

"No."

"Look," I said earnestly, "according to Chi Kung theory, the cause is simple. The flow of chi to your eyes is blocked; hence, your eyes cannot function properly. The therapeutic principle is also simple, though the actual process may not

be easy. Once we have cleared the blockage and restored the energy flow, your eyes will function again."

"I understand that, Sifu. What do you suggest I do?"

"Come to Malaysia immediately, and I'll try to clear the blockage."

"I can't. I'm now literally groping in the dark. I can't even leave my house."

As it was also not feasible for me to fly to Australia immediately, I made what many people would regard as an impossible suggestion.

"Jane, I'll do distant chi transmission. Listen carefully to my instructions. Do the chi flow exercise I have taught you every morning at seven o'clock. Visualize vital energy gently breaking through the blockage, flowing to your eyes, cleansing and nourishing them. Repeat that in the evening around six o'clock. Then at night at nine o'clock, go into deep meditation. Again visualize good, vital energy breaking through the blockage and nourishing your eyes. I'll transmit chi to you to help you do the cleansing. But I can't afford to send you chi every night. I'll transmit chi twice or three times a week during your nightly meditation at nine o'clock your time, but I won't tell you the actual days. Whenever you feel you have received my chi, make full use of it to break through the blockage."

What happened was what some people would call a miracle. In less than three months, Jane could see normally. This happened years ago, and there has been no relapse since. Her eye specialists were stunned. "This just couldn't happen," they said.

People thought I was crazy when I talked about distant *chi* transmission. To ascertain whether it was possible, a public experiment was carried out in 1989, and is described in Chapter 18.

### The Root Cause of Degenerative Diseases

Lau, Steven and Jane are just three out of hundreds of people who have had their so-called "incurable" diseases relieved after practicing Chi Kung with me or my students. For ethical reasons, their names have been changed, but their case histories are genuine. Some of the so-called "incurable" diseases that have been cured by practicing Chi Kung include: arthritis, rheumatism, insomnia, asthma, diabetes, ulcers, kidney failure, hypertension, sexual inadequacy, impotence, migraines, and cancer.

Some people might say that if Chi Kung is so good at curing diseases, then doctors will be redundant. This is of course not true. We greatly value the services of our doctors, and are fully aware that in many aspects conventional medicine is superior to Chi Kung therapy. (Incidentally many of my Chi Kung students are also medical doctors.) For example, if a patient suffers from an acute illness, then he should consult a conventional doctor, not a Chi Kung therapist. But in other cases, such as chronic and degenerative diseases, Chi Kung offers an excellent alternative.

We do not, of course, say that everyone suffering from these diseases will be cured by practicing Chi Kung. No responsible person, not even the best doctors, can guarantee that their patients will be cured, because recovery depends on many factors besides the actual treatment. But we can offer methods that many patients suffering from these diseases have found extremely useful. We have a very high recovery rate. Whether the methods work for you will depend on other factors too, such as whether you have practiced them correctly and regularly.

Can a general method of *chi* flow be used to cure a wide range of diseases? To those familiar with the concept of chemotherapy in conventional medicine, where a particular drug is used to cure a particular illness, overall treatment by means of a general method appears ridiculous. But it is not ridiculous; it is in fact logical and scientific if we understand the underlying principles.

It may surprise some people that all the diseases mentioned above have the same root cause—dysfunction of particular organs due to a blockage in the flow of *chi*. Indeed, the basic Chinese medical principle that if we cleanse the meridians to bring about a harmonious flow of *chi*, we can eliminate hundreds of illnesses, is a very concise statement of a great medical truth. Of course to those not familiar with Chinese medical philosophy, this basic principle appears ridiculous, just as the basic statement that everything—tadpole or mountain, table or elephant—is made of atoms may seem ridiculous to those not familiar with physics.

At all times and in all of us, fat is being deposited in our blood vessels, sugar is pouring into our blood stream, acid is accumulating in our stomachs, calcium is solidifying in our kidneys, pollutants are clogging our lungs, and toxic waste is choking our body cells. Yet we do not develop hypertension, diabetes, ulcers, kidney stones, asthma, or rheumatism so long as our bodies function naturally, so long as the elaborate system of *chi* flow (which corresponds to flow of electric impulses in Western medical thinking) feeds the necessary information to all parts of our bodies.

Our bodies are like gigantic biochemical plants, capable of producing all of the chemicals needed to neutralize excessive residues. But the parts of the body, the countless glands, must be fed the right information so that they know what to produce, and this is possible only when the flow of *chi* is uninterrupted and harmonious.

## *Meridians—the Pathways of Energy Flow*

The pathways of *chi* flow are called meridians. Some critics ask, "Where are the meridians? When a surgeon operates on a person, he does not find any meridians." They forget that the surgeon does not see air either, but it is still there.

It is useful to compare a meridian with a stream. A stream, unlike a pipe, has no defined boundary. It is simply where water flows, and it may constantly change its shape, although the change is so small that it generally maintains a definite line of flow. In the same way, a meridian has no fixed boundary. It exists where the *chi* flow is, though it maintains its general form.

Meridians (called *mai* in Chinese) are of two kinds: the main ones are called channels (*jing*), and the branches are called collaterals (*luo*). In many books, however, the term "meridians" is often used to denote channels, and that is the term I shall be using.

Meridians, or channels, can be classified into two groups: primary and secondary. Primary meridians are those that pass through internal organs; secondary meridians do not. There are twelve pairs of primary meridians flowing in a never-ending circle. For simplicity, only one of each pair is described. The twelve meridians are as follows:

1. Lung meridian
2. Colon meridian
3. Stomach meridian
4. Spleen meridian
5. Heart meridian
6. Intestine meridian
7. Urinary Bladder meridian
8. Kidney meridian
9. Pericardium meridian
10. Triple Warmer meridian
11. Gall Bladder meridian
12. Liver meridian

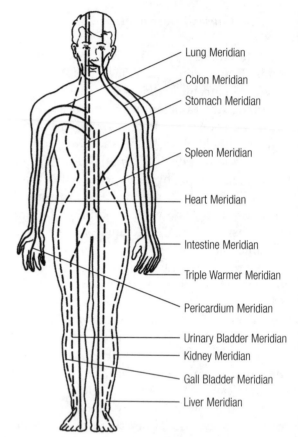

Lung Meridian
Colon Meridian
Stomach Meridian
Spleen Meridian
Heart Meridian
Intestine Meridian
Triple Warmer Meridian
Pericardium Meridian
Urinary Bladder Meridian
Kidney Meridian
Gall Bladder Meridian
Liver Meridian

*Fig. 4.1 The Twelve Primary Meridians*

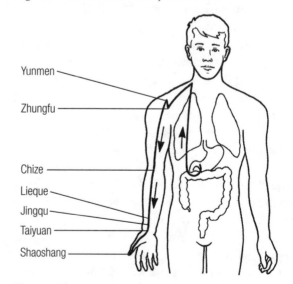

Yunmen
Zhungfu
Chize
Lieque
Jingqu
Taiyuan
Shaoshang

*Fig. 4.2 The Lung Meridian*

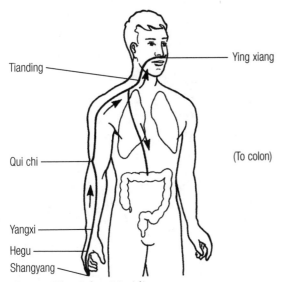

Fig. 4.3 The Colon Meridian

From each meridian there are countless branches and sub-branches. The locations of the twelve meridians are shown in a simplified form in *figure 4.1*.

Each of the twelve primary meridians is shown separately in *figures 4.2–4.13*. Their important energy points are also shown. An energy point, sometimes referred to as vital point, is where energy is focused or gathered. Where the focusing or gathering of energy is large, it is referred to as an energy field, which is similar to the Indian *chakra*.

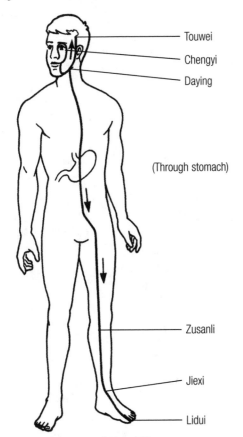

*Fig. 4.4 The Stomach Meridian*

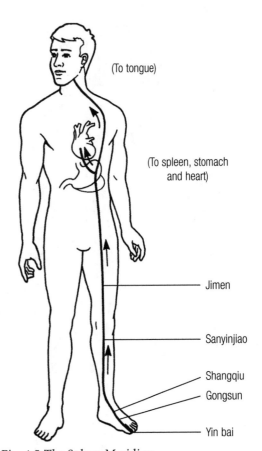

*Fig. 4.5 The Spleen Meridian*

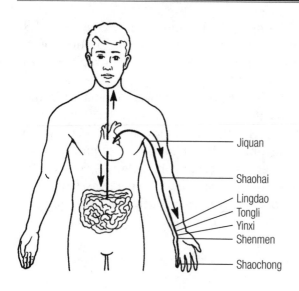

Jiquan

Shaohai

Lingdao
Tongli
Yinxi
Shenmen

Shaochong

*Fig. 4.6 The Heart Meridian*

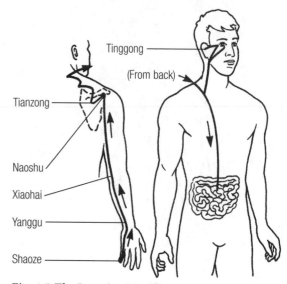

Tinggong

(From back)

Tianzong

Naoshu

Xiaohai

Yanggu

Shaoze

*Fig. 4.7 The Intestine Meridian*

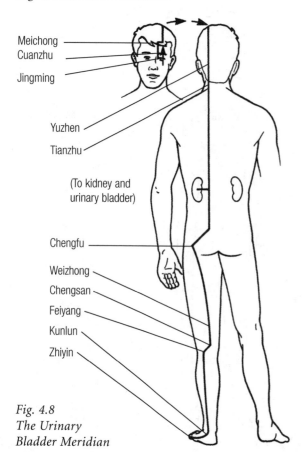

Meichong
Cuanzhu

Jingming

Yuzhen

Tianzhu

(To kidney and
urinary bladder)

Chengfu

Weizhong

Chengsan

Feiyang

Kunlun

Zhiyin

*Fig. 4.8
The Urinary
Bladder Meridian*

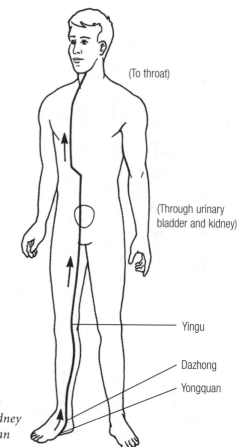

(To throat)

(Through urinary
bladder and kidney)

Yingu

Dazhong

Yongquan

*Fig. 4.9
The Kidney
Meridian*

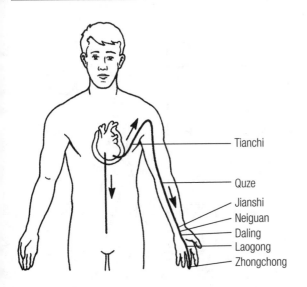

Fig. 4.10 The Pericardium Meridian

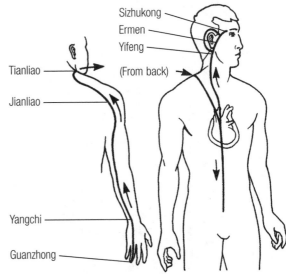

Fig. 4.10 The Triple Warmer Meridian

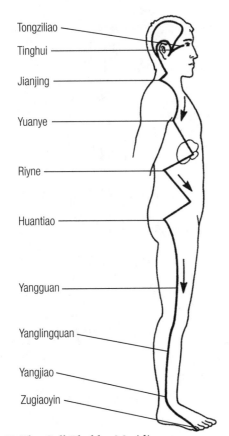

Fig. 4.12 The Gall Bladder Meridian

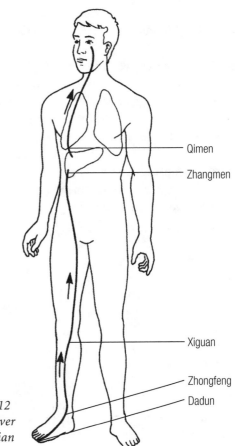

Fig. 4.12
The Liver
Meridian

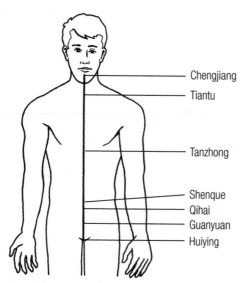

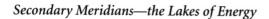

Fig. 4.14 The Ren or (Conceptual) Meridian

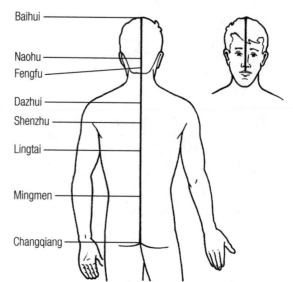

Fig. 4.15 The Du or (Governing) Meridian

### Secondary Meridians—the Lakes of Energy

Some classical writers referred to the primary meridians as energy streams, and the secondary meridians as energy lakes. Streams—because the primary meridians transport essential nutrients to every cell, and remove toxic waste from it. Lakes—because the secondary meridians serve as reservoirs, storing excess energy and using it to replenish the streams when the need arises.

There are eight secondary meridians, as follows:

1. *Ren mai* or conceptual meridian
2. *Du mai* or governing meridian
3. *Chong mai* or rushing meridian
4. *Dai mai* or belt meridian
5. *Yin qiao mai* or in-tall meridian
6. *Yang giao mai* or out-tall meridian
7. *Yin wei mai* or in-protective meridian
8. *Yang wei mai* or out-protective meridian

Of all the primary and secondary meridians, the two most important are the *ren* meridian and

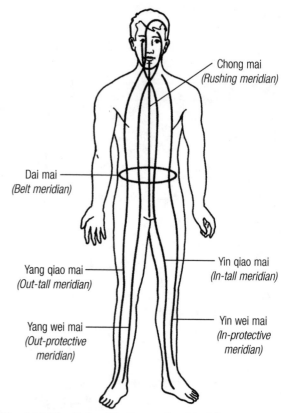

Fig. 4.16 The Other Six Seconadry Meridians

the *du* meridian. They are so important that the *ren* meridian is regarded as the sea of all *yin* energy, while the *du* meridian is the sea of all *yang* energy. *Ren* means conception, suggesting that energy flow starts from the *ren* meridian. *Du* means governing, suggesting that energy flow is controlled by the *du* meridian. Chi Kung masters throughout the ages have claimed that if one achieves a continuous flow of *chi* round the *ren* and *du* meridians, one will eliminate hundreds of illnesses. Experience shows that this is no exaggeration.

The *ren* and the *du* meridians are shown with their major energy points in *figures 4.14* and *4.15*.

The other six secondary meridians are shown in *figure 4.16*.

### Curing the Incurable with Chi Flow

*Induced Chi Flow* is a wonderful exercise for curing illness. One of the greatest physicians of all time, Hua Tuo, highly recommended this exercise as preventive medicine. There are three important points that any beginner should be aware of:

1. You will probably be very surprised at what you experience in the exercise.
2. This exercise is totally non-religious. What is involved is your own vital energy flowing inside you, making your body move, as if involuntarily. It is certainly not any outside force entering your body.
3. Should you start to move vigorously, gently tell yourself to slow down. Never, never panic. Always remain relaxed and calm.

Loosen your clothing. Ensure that the space you have chosen is safe for performing the exercise— away from sudden drops, sharp edges and pointed corners. Then follow these steps:

1. Stand relaxed and upright. Place your middle finger (left for men, right for women) on your navel and gently press about ten times. Then drop the finger to your side.
2. Use the other middle finger (right for men, left for women) to gently massage the *baihui* vital point, at the crown of your head, about five times. Then drop the finger to your side.
3. Perform *Lifting The Sky* (see Chapter 1) about 15–20 times. Each time you complete the sequence, pause for one or two seconds to feel *chi* flowing down your body.
4. Perform *Carrying The Moon* (see Chapter 2) about 15–20 times. Pause at the end of each sequence for one or two seconds to feel *chi* flowing down your body.
5. Stand relaxed with your eyes gently closed. If you are already swaying or moving, proceed to the next step. If not, then visualize a cascade of vital energy flowing from your head down your whole body. Enjoy the pleasant, tingling sensation, if you can feel it.
6. If you start to sway or move, follow the movements gently; do not go against them, as they are induced by *chi* flowing inside your body. After some time, the movements will become involuntary. Sometimes you may move from your position. You will find this experience very relaxing and enjoyable. Your eyes should be gently closed throughout. Later, when you are proficient in this exercise, you may open your eyes.
7. If you find that you are beginning to move vigorously, just tell yourself to slow down. If you find that the movements have suddenly become vigorous before you can do anything about it, do not worry. Remain calm, tell yourself to slow down, and you will do so. It is that simple. This exercise, incidentally, also illustrates that you can exercise mind over matter.

8.  After about ten minutes of *Induced Chi Flow* movements, or at any time when you want to stop, just tell your movements to stop. It is very important that you do *not* stop abruptly. Let your movements come to a graceful end.

9.  Remain still for a minute or two, with your eyes still closed. Then rub your palms together to warm them, and place them on your eyes as you open them. Massage your face gently. Then walk about briskly for about thirty steps.

This exercise is priceless. If you practice it consistently, it will prevent degenerative diseases, or start to cure them if you are already a sufferer.

# CHAPTER FIVE

# I Actually Live Twice—Through Chi Kung

> Through the centuries healing has been practiced by folk healers who are guided by a traditional wisdom that sees illness as a disorder of the whole person, involving not only the patient's body, but also his mind, his self-image, his dependence on the physical and social environment, as well as his relation to the cosmos.
>
> H.R.H. Prince Charles

## Prince's Advice and Emperor's Secret

The above advice, given by His Royal Highness Charles, Prince of Wales, to the British Medical Association in 1982, also sums up the basic philosophy of Chi Kung therapy. Chi Kung therapy sees illness as a disorder of the whole person, hence it treats the patient holistically, not just the diseased parts or the symptoms. It involves not only the physical body, but also the emotional, mental and spiritual aspects of the person; and it enhances his self-image as well as unifying him with the cosmos. *Induced Chi Flow* is an effective way to achieve all these aims.

*Induced Chi Flow* worked for thousands of years before modern medicine, though in the past it was often practiced exclusively by privileged people or selected disciples. Chinese records show that *Induced Chi Flow* was popularly practiced by emperors of the Qin, and the Han Dynasties. Han Wu Ti, the famous Martial Emperor of the Han Empire, owed his longevity to *Induced Chi Flow*.

*Induced Chi Flow* is a generic term referring to a class of Chi Kung movements whereby the practitioner moves involuntarily, owing to vital energy flowing inside his body as a result of appropriate physical and mental exercises. Generally the movements are gentle and graceful, but sometimes they may be vigorous. Sometimes the practitioners may actually shout and laugh, and roll about on the ground—something the uninitiated have to see to believe. I assure you, however, that what I am describing here is not merely something that has been recorded in classical Chi Kung texts, but is based on what actually happens in my Chi Kung classes.

## Five-Animal Play

Probably the best-known form of *Induced Chi Flow* is the *Five-Animal Play*, formalized by the great Chinese doctor, Hua Tuo, who lived between the second and third centuries AD It is called "five-animal" because the involuntary movements of the practitioner resemble movements of five animals—the tiger, the bear, the deer, the bird and the monkey.

For a time, because of inadequate under-standing, many people, including masters, thought that practitioners consciously imitated the movements of these animals. Indeed there are still many Chi Kung students who practice *Five-Animal Play* in this way.

But research in China reveals that the movements actually preceded the naming of them. The practitioners did not act consciously, but when they moved about *involuntarily* while in a Chi Kung trance, their movements were sometimes weird and animated. Some might jump about and frolic like a monkey; some make ferocious sounds like a tiger; others shape their fingers like antlers. Their movements were all different from one another, yet they could be grouped into five major categories, and past masters used the terms "tiger," "bear," "deer," "bird," and "monkey" to designate these categories. In other words, *Five-Animal Play* was devised not by consciously following the movements of five animals, but rather, that five animals were used to describe the involuntary movements of the practitioners while in a meditative Chi Kung state.

Frolicking like a monkey, shaping the fingers like a deer's antlers—I would not have believed it myself if I had not personally seen and experienced it! But actually, the movements do not necessarily resemble those of the five animals; the names are merely terms to classify the movements.

The first time these movements occurred in my Chi Kung class was when Percy, a young man of about thirty who suffered from arthritis, started hitting his body vigorously all over with his fists. Then he knelt down and performed some strange actions. Although I had earlier told the class that this might happen, most people were surprised when it did; some were scared, and a few thought that an evil spirit had entered Percy's body. But the most interesting aspect was that when Percy completed his antics about twenty minutes later, he told us that it was one of the most beautiful experiences he had ever had. Not long after that, his arthritis was cured. Percy continued to practice Chi Kung to quite an advanced level, and later he developed some useful psychic abilities.

In the *Induced Chi Flow* exercise described in the previous chapter, we used *Lifting The Sky* and *Carrying The Moon*. Other actions can also be used.

Most people sway gently like a graceful willow tree while performing *Induced Chi Flow*. Remember to use your mind to slow down your motions whenever they start to become too vigorous. If you do not slow yourself down, you may progress to movements, and sometimes sounds, that resemble those of the five animals. It is not advisable to allow your movements to become too vigorous initially, in case you lose control. As you become more familiar with the exercise, and more confident of your control, you may gradually allow yourself to move more energetically. Then, one day, you may find yourself roaring like a tiger or gamboling like a deer. But as you progress further, the movements usually become gentle again.

### Some Puzzling Questions on Induced Chi Flow

Why does our body seem to move involuntarily in a *chi* flow exercise, even though we are actually in full control? It is because we are so relaxed physically and mentally that the internal *chi* movements, which have been engendered by appropriate exercises, are expressed outwardly.

*Chi*, like blood, is flowing in our body all the time, though we are normally unaware of it. In the meditative Chi Kung state, our perception becomes more enhanced, and with Chi Kung exercises, our *chi* flow becomes more pronounced, enabling us to experience our body moving in unison with the internal flow of *chi*.

Why then, if we let ourselves go, may we frolic like a monkey, walk like a bear, roll on the floor, or perform other strange actions? According to Chinese medical philosophy, there are five different types of energy that correspond to our five "storage" organs: the heart, fiver, spleen, lungs and kidneys. These different energies behave differently.

For example, the heart energy, characterized by joy, is expressed through the tongue, and may make us chirp like a happy bird. The liver energy, characterized by anger, is expressed through the eyes, and may cause muscles to twitch, making us shape our fingers like antlers. The spleen energy, characterized by worry, is expressed through the mouth, and may cause us to make funny faces like a monkey. The lung energy, characterized by sorrow, is expressed through the nose, and may make us roar like a tiger. The kidney energy, characterized by fear, is expressed through the ears, and may straighten our skeletal structure, making us walk like a bear.

A thorough understanding of these different energies and their behavior, which can be expressed in the concepts of *yin-yang* and the *Five Elemental Processes,* is extremely useful to the Chi Kung therapist. For instance, by observing how a patient reacts in his *chi* flow movements, a master can get a good idea of his illness. If the patient has difficulty standing upright, he may have some sexual ailments; making him walk like a bear and strengthening his kidney energy (which is related to sexual vitality) may solve his problems.

Why do some people shout, laugh or make strange noises while performing their *chi* flow movements? This is because they are so emotionally relaxed in the meditative Chi Kung state that the pent-up emotions that have long been denied expression, possibly because of social conventions, are released. The roaring, giggling or other sounds are a form of emotional catharsis.

Some people hit themselves during their *chi* flow exercise. Why? It is not that they are punishing themselves; they are actually performing a form of self-therapy. Usually the hitting is involuntarily aimed at the diseased part or parts. Rolling on the floor serves a similar purpose. Sometimes they hit themselves quite hard, and onlookers may become concerned that they will hurt themselves. But when they have completed their exercise, they will probably tell you not only that their involuntary movements were not painful, but also that the pain they previously suffered because of their sickness has disappeared!

Let us now examine several related questions. Are these people in trance? Have they lost control of themselves? Have they been hypnotized? Or, most serious of all, are they possessed by some outside force? The answer to all these questions is a definite "no." They are not in a trance, in the sense of being dazed and unaware of what they are doing, though they are in a trance-like Chi Kung state. They are fully in control of themselves. Should they want to change or stop their actions at any time, they are able to do so. In my classes, there have been occasions when my students' movements during *Induced Chi Flow* would have been embarrassing at other times—things like dancing in an effeminate manner, wriggling like a snake, or laughing like a madman. In all cases, when they were later questioned, they answered that they were fully aware of their actions, yet they chose to continue because they enjoyed them.

Similarly, they have not been hypnotized, and they are certainly not possessed by any outside force. Their movements, which are relatively involuntary but which they can actually control if they wish, are the outward expression of their own vital energy flowing in their bodies.

### The Benefits of Induced Chi Flow

Why do we practice *Induced Chi Flow*? Here are a few good reasons:

1.  Many people have heard about *chi*, have even practiced Chi Kung, but have never consciously experienced what *chi* is. *Induced Chi Flow* is one of the most obvious ways to experience it.
2.  *Induced Chi Flow* is a wonderful form of deep relaxation. It is flowing meditation.
3.  *Induced Chi Flow* is an effective way to readjust energy levels in our bodies.
4.  *Induced Chi Flow* clears energy blockages, cleanses the body of toxic waste, and brings vital energy to all the cells of our body. It is an excellent form of preventive medicine.
5.  It is also an excellent way of curing disease, especially insidious disease, of which you may not even be aware, because it has not yet manifested itself outwardly.

It is now no longer a secret how Han Wu Ti, despite having three thousand wives and the myriad problems of an expanding empire, could live to a ripe old age. He practiced *Induced Chi Flow* daily.

Nowadays you do not have to be an emperor to enjoy the benefits of *Induced Chi Flow*. Indeed, it has enabled a number of my students to live twice.

### Living a Second Life

Ron was about seventy years old. His heart problem was so serious that after he had been in a specialist hospital for a long time, his doctor was honest enough to advise him to go home instead of wasting money on hospital treatment that was not helping. He could not attend my Chi Kung class; he could not even walk ten steps without falling. Most people thought he would die.

I asked his family to bring him to my Chi Kung class at Taiping, about 150 km from my house. I sat him on a chair. Watched by several of my students, I first opened several of his energy points, then channeled *chi* into him to gently massage his heart and clear his energy blockages. Soon he convulsed and made grunting sounds. The movements generated by *Induced Chi Flow* were quite vigorous, and caused some concern and even fear among the onlookers. When he completed the Chi Kung exercise about fifteen minutes later, he said the experience had been exhilarating.

I taught him some simple Chi Kung exercises to help him practice *Induced Chi Flow* at home, and arranged to transmit *chi* to him every alternate night. I went into meditation, saw him in my mind, and directed my *chi* to massage and nourish his heart. I did this for four weeks, resting myself in the third week to recharge myself, and he carried on his daily, *Induced Chi Flow* for six months. (Be warned, however. Serious heart patients are strongly advised *not* to attempt *Induced Chi Flow* without the supervision of a Chi Kung master.)

Ron is now clear of his heart problem. The most memorable thing to me was his answer when I asked him to confirm his recovery with his doctors. "I know I'm cured," he said. "I can do most things I used to do, though now with extra care and caution. Why should I seek confirmation from those who couldn't cure me in the first place? It may start my problem all over again!"

Another person who lives a second life because of Chi Kung is Margaret. She had cancer, mistakenly regarded by most people as an incurable, fatal disease. In fact there have been so many reports of authentic cures of cancer by "unorthodox" means, like meditation and faith healing, that some people rightly wonder why established research organizations have not studied these cures in detail.

Margaret, like many of my students suffering from cancer, recovered from this morbid disease by practicing Chi Kung. *Induced Chi Flow* is one of the major exercises they did. Margaret has practiced Chi Kung for more than two years now, and during this time she not only surprised her orthodox doctors with her cancer cure, but also relieved herself of other ailments like migraine, insomnia and nervousness.

It is interesting to note that cancer was not mentioned in classical Chinese medical texts. No one is sure whether this was because, although it existed, the ancient Chinese did not know about it, or whether it was because its incidence among the ancient Chinese was negligible. The nearest description to cancer they had was "poisonous growth," which they regarded as non-fatal and curable.

### A Simple Exercise That May Save Your Life

This exercise, called *Positive Visualization*, is so bafflingly simple that many people might question whether it works. In fact, not only has it worked wonders in my experience, but I can also explain its working scientifically.

Practice the exercise in a quiet, pleasant environment without distractions. Sit cross-legged in a standard meditation pose, or up-right on a seat, or lean back on a comfortable chair, or lie on a bed or a couch. Close your eyes and relax deeply. Then visualize your diseased part. Literally will it to recover—but do so gently. Hold the image of that part in the process of recovering (and later, recovered) as long as you can in your mind's eyes. Again, do this gently.

When you lose your image, rest your mind for a short while, still with your eyes closed. Then repeat the process. Practice the whole exercise for about five minutes at least twice a day for between three and eight months.

This process seems nonsensical if we still cling to the idea that man is a machine and illness is a disorder of parts of the machine. But if we see him according to the worldview derived from the latest discoveries of modern science, then it is both logical and natural. Since Bohr's Principle of Complementarity and Heisenberg's Principle of Uncertainty, scientists have accepted the fact that, at the subatomic level, the mind directly affects matter. Ancient masters of many great civilizations knew this great truth long ago.

At the subatomic and unconscious level, our bodies constantly cure and regenerate themselves. All the wear and tear inside our bodies, of which we are not aware, is constantly repaired in this natural way. Scientists have discovered that all the cells in our bodies are constantly being renewed at different rates, but that in seven months, there is a total turnover of our cells. In other words, the body you have now is totally different from the one you had seven months ago!

When the rate of self-curing and self-regeneration cannot match the rate of damage and injury, then illness surfaces. In the *Positive Visualization* exercise, we enhance our self-curing and self-regenerating ability. We also use our minds, as we hold the image of the recovery process, to direct our cells to be designed the way we want. This exercise is one efficient way to realize what Prince Charles said about involving the patient's self-image in the quotation at the beginning of this chapter. It is indeed amazing how much modern science is found in ancient wisdom.

# CHAPTER SIX

## *The Way to a Long and Healthy Life*

> Mediocre medicine cures diseases; superior medicine prevents them.
>
> *Nei Jing*

### Chi Kung as Preventive and Curative Medicine

Chinese medical philosophy has always emphasized the superiority of maintaining good health over curing illness. Chi Kung is preventive medicine *par excellence*. But it is even more: when you practice Chi Kung you experience at the same time both its preventive and its curative functions. If you have a disease, Chi Kung will cure it; if not, Chi Kung will promote your health and longevity. This preventive-cum-curative quality of Chi Kung makes it the unique healing system of the world.

It is natural to be healthy. It is only when certain parts of our bodies fail to function naturally that sickness occurs. The causes of dysfunction may be exopathogenic, organic, or psychosomatic.

Exopathogenic agents, like bacteria and viruses, are always present in our bodies, but they are kept in check (sometimes even exploited to do useful work for us) as long as our bodies function naturally. Toxins are continually clogging our organs, but as long as we function naturally, these toxins will be neutralized by the chemicals produced by our body. Our minds (or brains, as some neurosurgeons may insist) are continually stressed, but again, if nature runs its course, we will be adequately relieved after sleep and rest.

The Chinese concept of health is also wider than that of the West. To be healthy is not just to be free from disease. A person cannot be called healthy if he is often restless, irritable or extremely forgetful, cannot concentrate or sleep soundly, and has no zest for work or play.

How does Chi Kung promote health? First, it frees us from disease; it prevents as well as cures illness. Then it helps us to grow emotionally, mentally and spiritually, giving us the wonderful benefits of health in its wider sense. In this chapter we will study the preventive and curative qualities of Chi Kung in promoting our physical, and emotional health, leaving the mental and spiritual aspects to subsequent chapters. For those who are used to conventional Western medical concepts, the following explanation may resemble an exciting journey to exotic new worlds.

### Cleansing Meridians and Balancing Yin-Yang

Although the details of Chinese medical philosophy can be complex and puzzling, fundamentally, the how's and why's of Chi Kung therapy, as well as of other branches of Chinese medicine, can be reduced to two simple principles: the cleansing of meridians to achieve harmonious energy flow, and the restoration of *yin-yang* balance.

*Yin-yang* is probably the most widely used, and most misunderstood, concept in Chinese medicine. Many Western authors have given the impression that the Chinese regard *yin* and *yang* as the two basic ingredients or forces of which the universe is composed. This is quite wrong. *Yin* and *yang* are not absolute units; they are merely symbolic terms, and as symbols, they may mean different things at different times.

*Yin* and *yang* refer to the two opposing yet complementary aspects of everything in the universe, from concrete objects to abstract ideas. They are relative to each other, and each exists because of the other. Take a simple concept like big and small. We say an elephant is big because we usually compare it to a smaller object, like a mouse or a human. If we compare an elephant to a mountain, then the elephant is very small.

Let us now examine a more abstract idea: say courage and cowardice. Just as with big and small, courage is relative to cowardice; it exists because of cowardice, and vice versa. For example, if someone climbs a cliff but only gets half way, some people might consider it cowardly not to get to the top. However, for someone who suffers from vertigo, climbing over half way is an act of courage.

In both cases, we refer to one aspect, small or cowardly, as *yin*, and the other aspect, big or courageous, as *yang*. Can we reverse the terms, by referring to small and cowardly as *yang*, and big and courageous as *yin*? We can, but we may cause some problems because by convention whatever is negative, feminine, dark, cold, yielding, below, inside, or structural, is referred to as *yin*, and their counterparts as *yang*.

### The Yin-Yang of Contagious Diseases

The Chinese refer to the body's natural self-defense system as *yin*, and all exopathogenic agents as *yang*. Although at any one time, there are millions of germs in our bodies—many of them actually deadly—we are not sick, because our *yin* defense can balance the *yang* exopathogenic agents. If this *yin-yang* balance is disturbed, then illness may occur. For example, if the *yin* defense is weakened, perhaps by anxiety or fatigue, then we may fall sick even if the number or potency of *yang* exopathogenic agents has not increased. This *yin-yang* disharmony is caused by insufficient *yin*.

On the other hand, the *yin* defense may remain constant but the exopathogenic agents increase substantially, such as when we take contaminated food or breathe in an excessive number of harmful germs. Then illness may occur, and this *yin-yang* disharmony is caused by excessive *yang*. How does Chi Kung prevent or cure contagious diseases? When disease-causing microorganisms attack certain parts of the body, reserve energy is channeled to meet these attacks. But if the meridians are blocked, then the flow of reserve energy is hindered, and illness results.

When we practice Chi Kung we cleanse our meridians, harmonizing energy levels and promoting a smooth flow of reserve energy to the areas under attack, thus restoring the *yin-yang* balance. Moreover, practicing Chi Kung increases our reserves of energy, thus preventing any possible outbreak of illness.

Research carried out in China recently using Western scientific apparatus has verified this. For example, a series of experiments carried out at Tientsin Chinese Medical Research Center on sixty-eight patients showed that the proportion of white blood cells, which are responsible for the body's self-defense, increased from an average of 57.7 percent to 78.1 percent after practicing Chi Kung for three months.[2] Experiments carried out at Jiangsu Chinese Medical Research Center showed that the amount of the antibody IgA, which is important for humoral immunity, increased from 767.5 mg percent to 1193.4 mg percent after three months of Chi Kung practice. The proportion of T-cells, which are important for cell-mediated immunity, was found to be 74.9 percent among Chi Kung practitioners, compared to 65.6 percent in other people.[3]

So practicing Chi Kung greatly enhances our immune system. When we can successfully prevent outbreaks of contagious diseases, we not only add to the quality of our lives now, but also give ourselves the opportunity to live more fully our natural life span.

## Clearing Dirt and Repairing Damage

Chi Kung's forte is in preventing and curing organic or degenerative diseases. All our vital organs are constantly toxified by pollutants and residues—cholesterol choking the heart, nitrites clogging brain cells, acid pouring into the stomach, calcium forming in the kidneys. But we are by nature able to detoxify ourselves, so long as our feedback systems function properly.

But if there is a blockage in our meridians, along which energy carrying vital information flows, then the efficiency of our feedback system will be affected. For example, if the set of meridians flowing from the heart to the central nervous system—the *yin* meridians—do not carry the right information regarding the amount of excessive cholesterol deposited there, or if the reverse set of meridians from the central nervous system to the heart—the *yang* meridians—do not carry the right instruction regarding the amount of hormones to be produced, then cardiovascular diseases may occur. The same principle applies to all other organs.

The cause of such organic or degenerative diseases is the blocking of energy, which disrupts the harmony of the *yin* and *yang* sets of meridians of the respective organs. Once the blockage is cleared, and the *yin-yang* balance restored, the disease will disappear as a matter of course.

Practicing Chi Kung keeps all our vital organs in their proper forms and functions, cleansing them of dirt and repairing damage as soon as they occur, giving them no chance to develop into and manifest as organic or degenerative diseases. This is one of the ways in which Chi Kung enhances quality of life and promotes longevity.

## Energy Flow for Emotional Stability

The third group of diseases mentioned above is psychosomatic, which is described by the Chinese, if they ever make such arbitrary classifications, as emotional illness.

In the previous chapter, we mentioned that the five vital organs—heart, liver, spleen, lungs and kidneys—are related to the five basic emotions, respectively joy, anger, worry, sorrow and fear. A blockage of the flow of liver energy, for example, may cause it to be excessive, or *yang*, making the person easily prone to anger; conversely, a person who frequently becomes angry will damage his liver system.

The liver meridian flows into the lung meridian. A blockage in the flow of liver energy, therefore, may cause a deficiency of lung energy. This *yin* deficiency in the lung meridian may make the person unable to bear grief.

Further, according to the Chinese concept of the *Five Elemental Processes* (which will be explained in the next chapter), the liver, system, which corresponds to the Wood Process, directly affects the heart system, which corresponds to the Fire Process. "Too much Wood will cause excessive Fire," states a Chinese medical axiom. In simple language, this means a person who becomes easily angry will also harm his heart.

This may seem complicated, but imbalances are actually quite easily remedied by Chi Kung therapy. Cleanse the meridians and restore the *yin-yang* balance, and health will be restored. You will now be able to appreciate why Chinese medical philosophy emphasizes curing the patient, not just the disease. This may also suggest some reasons why at times Western doctors cannot find the cause of a disease, even though they and their patients know that it is real.

If, basing your ideas on Western medical philosophy, you are tempted to dismiss this organ-emotion correspondence or *Five Elemental Processes* as nonsensical, remember that Chinese medical philosophy is based on a different worldview. Asking a Chinese physician how he knows that blocking the liver energy arouses the emotion of anger is like asking a Western surgeon how he knows that an excess of nitrites in cranial nerves causes headaches. The Western surgeon might say, "Well, if when a patient complained of headaches I were to cut open his head and tear apart his cranial nerves, I would find excessive amounts of nitrites in them." The Chinese physician might reply, "If, when my patient is angry, I feel his pulse, I will find that his liver meridian is blocked."

The surgeon might further say, "If I were to cut open his cranial nerves to remove the excess nitrites, his headache would go, but he would probably go too. So I give him a painkiller instead, to numb his nerves so that he will not feel the headache even though it is actually still there." The Chinese physician will say, "If I press certain energy points to stop certain energy flows, the patient will not feel the anger, though it will still be there, as the liver energy is still blocked. So instead, I release the blockage. Then he will stop being angry, because the emotion of anger has been flushed out."

In other words, according to Chinese medical thinking, the cause of anger and other negative emotions is internal. For example, if you become angry because a waiter snatches away your unfinished meal while you turn aside to talk to a friend, it is not because of the action itself, but because that action generates a series of reactions inside your body that block the flow of your liver energy. If there is no energy blockage, then the action will not make you angry. You might even joke with the waiter asking whether you could pay only a portion of the bill because you have not finished the meal!

If your meridians are properly cleansed and your various organ-energies are flowing harmoniously, you will not harbor negative emotions, such as the inability to feel joy, a tendency to anger, unnecessary worrying, depression, and unreasonable fear. If you can appreciate this principle of organ-emotion correspondence, you will understand why stressful living can cause so much sickness related to internal organs. On a positive note, you will understand why Chi Kung masters, whose organ-energies are flowing harmoniously, are not only fit and healthy, but also calm and joyful, even under trying circumstances. They are, therefore, in a better position to live long, satisfying lives.

### Empty Your Heart, Fill Your Abdomen

To cleanse our meridians and balance *yin-yang*, we need energy. One of the best ways to obtain this energy is to, "empty your heart, fill your abdomen"—a Chi Kung technique known more prosaically as *Abdominal Breathing*.

If you are used to chest breathing, it is difficult to change to *Abdominal Breathing* immediately. But the following method can make the technique easier.

Stand upright and relaxed with your feet fairly close together. Place one hand on your middle energy field, about two inches below your navel. Place your other hand over it. Open your mouth slightly. Then empty your heart—that is, dispel irrelevant thoughts. It is important to have an "empty heart" throughout this exercise.

With both palms, gently press your abdomen in

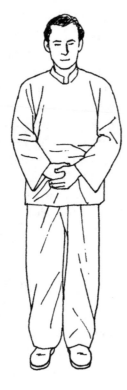

*Fig. 6.1 Abdominal Breathing*

about 10–20 times, drop your hands to your sides and stand still with your eyes closed for about five minutes. Practice this twice daily for at least two weeks before proceeding to the next stage.

For the second stage, repeat the same movements as in stage 1, but as you press your abdomen, gently visualize bad *chi* (or negative energy) flowing from your abdomen up your body and out of your mouth. Practice this stage for at least two weeks before going on to the next one, gradually increasing the counts when pressing and releasing your abdomen, but keeping the holding time to two counts.

In the third stage, the movements are the same, but as you release your abdomen, gently visualize good cosmic energy flowing through your nose, down your body and filling your abdomen. In other words, as you press your abdomen, bad *chi* flows out; as you release it, good *chi* flows in. Do not worry about your breathing; let it be natural. As before, stand still for about five minutes with an "empty heart" when you have finished.

one smooth continuous movement for four counts (about four seconds). Make sure that you do not breathe in as you press your abdomen. Hold that position for two counts. Then release the pressure of your palms in one smooth, continuous movement for four counts, thus allowing your abdomen to return to its original position. Hold for two counts.

This process—pressing, holding, releasing, holding—constitutes one breathing unit, or one breath, and it takes ten counts (about ten seconds). Start with ten breaths for each practice session, and gradually increase by one or two breaths. Do not worry about your breathing yet. At this stage, it will be natural or spontaneous, but remember not to breathe in as you press your abdomen.

After pressing and releasing your abdomen

*Fig. 6.1 Abdominal Breathing*

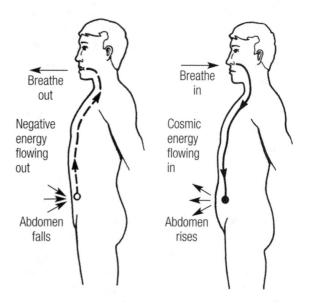

Proceed to stage four only after you have practiced the preliminary stages for at least six weeks. This is the "empty your heart, fill your abdomen" stage proper.

Empty your mind of all irrelevant thoughts. Breathe out gently through your mouth as you gently press your abdomen to let out bad *chi*, and breathe in gently through your nose as you release your abdomen to let good cosmic *chi* flow in. Perform this *Abdominal Breathing* for thirty-six breaths. Then continue with *Standing Meditation* for about five to fifteen minutes.

During the *Standing Meditation*, you may use *Positive Visualization* (described in the previous chapter) to solve any health problem you may have. *Abdominal Breathing*, combined with *Standing Meditation* and *Positive Visualization*, is a powerful technique for curing illness. But it takes time. If you are prepared to practice daily for six months, your doctor will probably be surprised to see you so full of health and vitality.

Albert, a good friend of Jane, whom I referred to in Chapter 4, accompanied her to Malaysia when she came to thank me for restoring her eyesight. For three years, he had suffered from a viral chest infection, which his doctor considered incurable. More to please Jane than anything else, Albert practiced the *Abdominal Breathing* and *Positive Visualization* I taught him.

When I visited Australia a few months later, Jane told me:

"You know, Sifu, Albert the Skeptic is now cured of his so-called incurable chest infection. He found out in a most interesting way. When he went for his regular check-up, he said to his doctor, 'I think I'm all right now. I haven't had any problems with my chest lately.' 'Don't be naive,' his doctor said. 'Your chest infection cannot be cured. I'll show you.' So he took out Albert's X-ray plates to show him where the infections were. But he couldn't find any. After a long while, he turned to Albert. 'Yes,' he said, 'I think you are cured!'"

# CHAPTER SEVEN

# Chi Kung for Stress Management and Mental Illness

And what is there to life if a man cannot hear the lonely cry of the whip-poor-will or the arguments of the frogs around a pond at night? I am a red man and do not understand. The Indian prefers the soft sound of the wind darting over the face of a pond, and the smell of the wind itself, cleansed by a midday rain, or scented with the pinon pine. The air is precious to the red man, for all things share the same breath—the beast, the tree, the man, they all share the same breath.

Native American Indian Chief Seattle, 1854

### The Joy of a Stress free Life

How many of us can still appreciate the soft sound of the wind darting over the face of a pond, or the smell of the wind itself, cleansed by the midday rain, or scented with the pinon pine? Not many, as most of us today are preoccupied with stress.

Stress, most doctors agree, is presently the number one troublemaker, causing both physical and mental illness as well as loss of efficiency for "healthy" people. The three most widely prescribed drugs in the world today all deal with stress.

Chi Kung is an excellent way to manage stress, as well as cure illnesses caused by stress—without the use of tranquillizers, antidepressants, surgery, or psychotherapy.

Experts have classified the factors that cause stress, or stressors as they are called, into three groups: major events, like bereavement and divorce; daily hassles, like traffic jams and provocative arguments; and continuing problems, like managerial responsibilities and occupational hazards. Events in these three groups generate strong emotions like grief, anger and anxiety which, if severe and unchecked, may lead to physical illness, especially degenerative diseases like ulcers, kidney stones, coronary disease and cancer; or to mental disorders, like phobias, neurasthenia, hypochondria, drug addiction, and schizophrenia.

While the West clearly distinguishes between physical and mental illness, and between disorders of the mind and of the brain, the Chinese do not have such distinctions because they have always regarded the patient as a whole person. What the West refers to as neurotic and psychotic diseases may be described by the Chinese as illnesses of the emotions or the mind (which the Chinese often call the heart). The distinction between emotional and mental sickness is vague.

Although psychiatrists never existed as a professional group in China, the standard of Chinese psychiatry is exceedingly high. Indeed, Western neuroscientists and psychiatrists would benefit tremendously if they cared to study the philosophy and practice of the Chinese in this field.

## Emotional Diseases are Best Cured by Emotions

The Chinese have a saying that emotional diseases are best cured by emotions. As most mental illness is caused by negative emotions, Chinese physicians through the ages have frequently used the interplay of emotions, and nothing else, to cure mental diseases. Numerous interesting case histories have been recorded and the following is an example.

As Li Xian Da had done very well in an imperial civil service examination, the Emperor called him to the capital to become a deputy minister. His father became overexcited. First he laughed to himself many times a day, then he laughed incessantly, and later he became hysterical with laughter. No doctors could cure him of this peculiar disease. Li wanted to resign and go home. When the Emperor heard about it, he asked his imperial physician to cure Li's father.

"Your Majesty," said the physician, "no medicine can cure the senior Mr. Li of such a peculiar disease." When Li Xian Da heard this, he broke down. "But that doesn't mean he can't be cured," the physician added. "I'm quite sure I can cure him if your Majesty would allow me to play a little joke."

A few days later a troop of soldiers surrounded old Mr. Li's house and arrested his family. The general, who had come especially from the capital, shouted at him angrily: "You and Li Xian Da have plotted against the Emperor! I am here to execute you and your family."

Li was terrified. The first day in his cell, he was speechless and trembling with fear. The second day he wailed and howled. But on the third day he regained his senses, and was able to cry out that he and his son were innocent. Then the general released him and his family, and told them it was just a joke the imperial physician had suggested to cure his strange illness.

The imperial physician had applied the principle of "water destroys fire" to cure the hysterical laughing. To understand this principle, and how Chinese physicians use emotions to treat mental diseases, let us examine the concept of the *Five Elemental Processes.*

## The Five Elemental Processes

Although this principle is not as universally known in the West as the *yin-yang* concept, it is nevertheless used extensively in Chinese philosophy, medicine, military strategy, divination, astrology, alchemy, geomancy and other fields. The concepts of *yin-yang* and the *Five Elemental Processes*, known as *wu xing*, are often used to complement each other.

In Western literature, these *Five Elemental Processes* are frequently mistranslated as five elements, giving the impression that the Chinese consider them to be the basic ingredients of the universe. This is wrong. They do not refer to the composition of the universe, but to the behavior of processes.

Of course, there are countless processes in the universe, but ancient masters observed that they can all be grouped into five archetypes. Each archetype has its own typical pattern of behavior, and the ancient masters called them: metal, water, wood, fire and earth.

The masters also noticed that when processes interact with each other, they affect one another in characteristic ways. They summarized these archetypical behavior patterns as the principles of inter-creativity and inter-destructivity. Most books explain inter-creativity as, "metal creates water," "water creates wood," "wood creates fire," "fire creates earth," and "earth creates metal," thus forming a never-ending circle, as in *figure 7.1.*

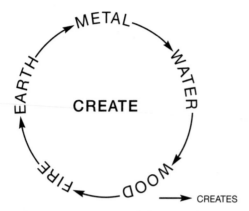

Fig. 7.1 The Inter-creativity of the Five Elemental
Processes

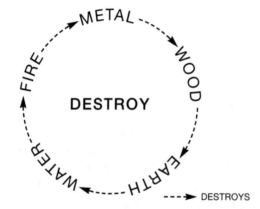

Fig. 7.2 The Inter-destructivity of the Five Elemental
Processes

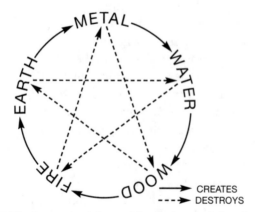

Fig. 7.3 The Inter-creativity and Inter-destructivity of
the Five Elemental Processes

Similarly, inter-destructivity is explained as "metal destroys wood," "wood destroys earth," "earth destroys water," "water destroys fire," "fire destroys metal," again forming a continuous circle, as in *figure 7.2*. The combination of creativity and inter-destructivity is shown in *figure 7.3*.

To most people, including the Chinese, the real problem of understanding the *Five Elemental Processes* begins when this explanation ends. Nevertheless, we shall have a better idea of these five processes if we translate the symbols into examples.

Dissemination of knowledge, for example, is regarded as a water process, because the water process, among other things, is concerned with spreading. When knowledge is made available to more people, it will lead to their advancement, which is a wood process, as the wood process is concerned with growth. This can be expressed symbolically as "water creates wood." In more universal terms, it means that processes that spread generally promote growth. Another example of this "water creates wood" principle is that when Chi Kung is more widely practiced, the health of the world's people will be improved.

Continued advancement will lead to a conflict of interests, which is a fire process, be cause the fire process is concerned with activity. Hence, "wood creates fire." However, if knowledge is well disseminated, it may prevent conflict; hence "water destroys fire."

If there is conflict, people of similar interests will join forces, which is an earth process, as the earth process is concerned with coming together. This is "fire creates earth." On the other hand, earth is destroyed by wood. For example, when people's prosperity is increasing, they may not come together even though they have similar interests.

When people come together, they will discuss,

which is regarded as a metal process, as the metal process is concerned with resonance. This is symbolized as "earth creates metal." But if these people are in conflict, then the discussion may not be fruitful, which is "fire destroys metal."

Fruitful discussion will lead to the spread of knowledge, which is "metal creates water." But if the people entrusted with the dissemination of knowledge concentrate in one place instead of dispersing, then the spread of knowledge is hampered. This is "earth destroys water."

This is of necessity only a simple example of the principle; other aspects, like excessiveness and inadequacy, which may cause anomalous results,

cannot be covered here. Nevertheless, the above explanation provides some idea of how the concept of the *Five Elemental Processes* can be used to cure mental illness.

### Elemental Processes in Emotional Interplay

The concept of the five elemental processes, or *wu xing*, is applicable to everything from subatomic particles to distant stars. From their long years of observation, great masters have bequeathed to us appropriate classifications of many common phenomena. The most useful ones for medicine are listed in *figure 7.4*.

*Fig. 7.4 Mutual Correspondence of the Five Elemental Process*

| | WOOD | FIRE | EARTH | METAL | WATER |
|---|---|---|---|---|---|
| **SEASONS** | Spring | Summer | Late Summer | Autumn | Winter |
| **DIRECTIONS** | East | South | Center | West | North |
| **CLIMATIC CONDITIONS** | Wind | Heat | Dampness | Dryness | Cold |
| **ZHANG ORGANS** | Liver | Heart | Spleen | Lungs | Kidneys |
| **FU ORGANS** | Gall Bladder | Intestines | Stomach | Colon | Urinary Bladder |
| **SENSE ORGANS** | Eyes | Tongue | Mouth | Nose | Ears |
| **EMOTIONS** | Anger | Joy | Worry | Sorrow | Fear |
| **COLORS** | Green | Red | Yellow | White | Black |
| **TASTES** | Sour | Bitter | Sweet | Tart | Salty |
| **SOUNDS** | Call | Laugh | Sing | Cry | Moan |

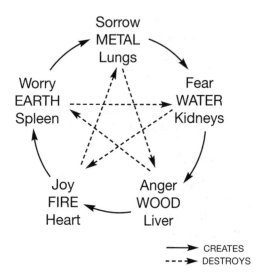

Fig. 7.5 Organ-Emotion Correspondence

If we pick out from this table the information concerning our vital organs and basic emotions, we can devise a diagram like *figure 7.5*.

Using this simple diagram (which symbolizes profound truths which have taken Chinese scientists centuries to evolve); we can use the interplay of emotions to cure emotional sickness. For example, the imperial physician in the story above used fear to overcome joy. Li senior became so frightened that his fear overcame the illness caused by excessive joy. In the previous chapter, we mentioned that a person who is easily angered will harm his heart. This can be seen from the diagram—excessive wood creates excessive fire, which will burn the heart. If a patient's mental illness is the result of excessive worry, we may cure him by making him very angry; or if he suffers from excessive anger, we can help by taking him to a tragic play.

What does all this emotional interplay have to do with *chi*? Everything! Because, as we have seen in the previous chapter, emotional problems are caused by energy blockages in the respective meridians.

*Chi* forms the very basis of Chinese medicine. Whether in diagnosis, prognosis, therapeutics, pathology, physiology, psychology or pharmacology, the fundamental factor is *chi*. This is sensible and logical, because we are, after all, actually bodies of *chi*.

A person becomes ill because, at the cellular level, his harmonious energy flow is disturbed. Chi Kung is an excellent way to correct this disturbed condition; other ways include acupuncture, herbal medicine and massage therapy.

### The Contrast between Western Treatment and Chi Kung

It is worth comparing how Western medicine and Chi Kung treat mental disorders. The three standard Western treatments for neurosis and psychosis are drugs, psychotherapy and electroconvulsive therapy.

Instead of drugs, which merely alleviate the symptoms, Chi Kung uses internal energy flow, which flushes out the repressed emotion. Instead of psychotherapy, which attempts to dress up an unacceptable situation so that it appears less unpleasant, Chi Kung uses meditation, which develops the patient's mind so that the enlarged mental capacity can now accept the previously unacceptable situation.

In electroconvulsive therapy, a small electric current is briefly applied to the patient, and it often causes unpleasant side effects like temporary memory loss. In Chi Kung, cosmic energy is channeled into the patient by a master, or "breathed" in from the universe by the patient himself, with tremendous benefits and no side-effects.

One great advantage Chi Kung has over Western treatments for mental illness is that the effects of Chi Kung are preventive as well as curative. Moreover, they are holistic; the same Chi Kung exercises are as beneficial for mental problems as for other forms of illness.

In other words, one does not have to be mentally ill to practice those Chi Kung exercises which are effective for curing mental sickness because they not only manage stress, thus preventing possible mental diseases, but can also cure or prevent physical illness.

### Chi Kung Treatment for Mental Illness

*Dao yin* exercises like *Lifting The Sky* and *Carrying The Moon* are effective for progressive relaxation. They also lead to *Induced Chi Flow*, which readjusts the body's energy levels, and flushes out repressed emotions, especially if we move vigorously and make strange sounds. (Our family and friends should be informed beforehand that these animated antics and sounds are not *expressions* of mental disorders, but the *means to get rid* of them.)

*Positive Visualization* can be used to correct our self-image—internally to ourselves and externally to others. For example, we can hold in our mind's eye a vision of ourselves free of phobia, depression or personality disorders. This exercise is difficult, however, and not advisable for those with severe mental illnesses. They should practice meditation to strengthen their minds before attempting this visualization exercise.

*Abdominal Breathing* is very helpful in cleansing the body of negative energies and replacing them with good cosmic energy. As you breathe out, think of your anxiety, obsession or any mental disorders being dispelled. If you are religious, you can think of God's grace, according to your own religious beliefs, flowing into you as you breathe in. Those with serious mental illnesses should practice *dao yin* and *chi* flow exercises to readjust their energy levels, and practice deep relaxation to

calm their minds, before attempting *Abdominal Breathing with Visualization*.

Betty suffered from schizophrenia for three years. She told me that she was the Virgin Mary come to this world to save mankind. At other times she told me that many religious figures were sinners, and that she herself might be some satanic force impersonating Virgin Mary.

I taught her *Lifting The Sky* and *Carrying The Moon*. I also opened some of her energy points to enhance her *Induced Chi Flow*. I told her to think of God's grace when she did *Standing Meditation*. The most difficult part was to persuade her to practice regularly. But now, two years later, she is no longer on drugs, she is surer of herself, seldom depressed, and can mix with her friends.

### Chi Kung Relaxation for Managing Stress

The following is a simple but effective method for managing stress. It is particularly useful to busy professionals and executives who feel fatigued or stressful in the midst of their work. Break off for five minutes to do this exercise, and you will be refreshed. Those who suffer from mental disorders will find the deep relaxation of this exercise a helpful preliminary for later curative techniques, like *chi* flow and *Abdominal Breathing*.

Lie down comfortably on a bed or couch, or lean back in a comfortable chair. Place your hands effortlessly at your sides, or on the armrests. Close your eyes gently and clear your mind of all thoughts. Smile from inside your heart.

Take three deep breaths slowly and gently. If you can breathe from your abdomen, do so; if not, breathe naturally. Gently follow the three deep, slow breaths with your mind. Then forget about your breathing. Tell yourself that you are going to enjoy deep relaxation for five minutes, and will come out of this meditation fresh and calm. (If you suffer from insomnia, tell yourself to have sweet sleep throughout the night and wake up fresh early next morning. Your insomnia may disappear before you realize it!) When you feel that five minutes is over, rub your palms, place them on your eyes as you open them, massage your face, and you will feel fresh and calm. It is that simple, but the benefits, over a period of time, are marvelous.

At first, you may find that what you thought was five minutes is only one or two. But as you progress, you will find that you come out of meditation exactly on time!

# PART THREE

# Vitality for Sport, Sex, and Youthfulness

# CHAPTER EIGHT

# Chi Kung for Sportsmen and Champions

If you watch a game, it's fun. If you play it, it's recreation. If you work at it, it's golf.

Bob Hope

### The Role of Chi Kung in Making Champions

All sports, whether golf or boxing, football or dancing, need energy and good judgment. Chi Kung supplies both these qualities. Just fifty years ago, China, despite her large population and long history, was unknown in international sports, but now she produces world champions, ranging from table tennis and badminton to gymnastics and swimming. The Chinese, who are generally small, have even broken world records in high jump and weightlifting.

What has made them progress so fast? One significant factor is Chi Kung. It is now an open secret that every Chinese team must have the service of at least one Chi Kung master, who not only uses Chi Kung therapy to help sportsmen recover from their injuries surprisingly fast, but also channels *chi* to them to enhance their performance.

The earliest modern Chinese attempt to apply Chi Kung to international sports with outstanding results was by the Chinese swimmer, Mu Xiang Xiong, who three times broke the world record for the 100 meter breast stroke in

1958 and 1959. Many readers will be surprised that his two basic Chi Kung exercises, meditation and the *Horse-riding Stance*, seem so unrelated to swimming; but these exercises actually provided him with a foundation of visualization, deep breathing, and strong legs, which was crucial in his competitions. In explaining how he applied the skills he had acquired in Chi Kung to his swimming, he said, "Each time I breathed in and out, I thought of each word in succession of the sentence: 'I'll break the one hundred meter world record.' Then I developed deep breathing until I could swim one hundred meters in only three breaths."[4]

Chi Kung was found to be so effective in enhancing sporting achievements that in 1978 the Chinese National Sports Council instructed selected specialized sport colleges to seriously study applying Chi Kung to sports.[5]

Energy is the basic requirement for any sportsman who wishes to excel, and Chi Kung, being an art that specifically develops energy, is obviously of great help. How does Chi Kung provide abundant energy? Let us learn a lesson from a child.

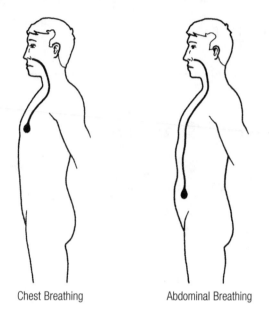

Chest Breathing          Abdominal Breathing

*Fig. 8.1 Contrast of Energy Flow in Chest Breathing and Abdominal Breathing*

### Learning a Lesson from a Child

If you play with a child, unless you are a trained athlete, you will probably be panting after a few minutes while the tiny tot is still bouncing with energy. What is the secret of the child's supply of energy?

If you observe how he breathes, you will get the answer. Every child breathes with his abdomen. That is the natural way of breathing, the way we all "breathed" when we were in our mother's womb. Top-class sportsmen, singers, martial artists and others who need an abundant supply of energy use *Abdominal Breathing* too.

*Figure 8.1* gives a visual explanation why *Abdominal Breathing* provides more energy. The flow of energy to the abdomen is much longer than that to the chest. Throat breathing, used by many elderly people, is worse. The flow of energy to the throat is so short that the person involved easily becomes short of breath.

A well-known surgeon who learned Chi Kung from me once raised an illuminating question. "How do we breathe into our abdomens?" he asked. "Our lungs are airtight: there is no way at all for air breathed in through the nose to reach the abdomen. Yet when I do *Abdominal Breathing*, I can clearly feel something in my abdomen."

I replied that what we breathe in is not just air, but also cosmic energy, and it is the cosmic energy that is felt at the abdomen. The ball of cosmic energy we feel at the abdomen, however, does not all come from the air we breathe; what we take in with each breath is just a small portion added to the energy already accumulated there.

An advanced Chi Kung practitioner can go further than *Abdominal Breathing*. He can send his breathing round the body, along the circle of the *ren* and *du* meridians, in what is called *Small Universal Chi Flow*, or *Micro-cosmic Energy Flow*. *Figure 8.2* shows the *chi* flow in the *Small Universe* or *Micro-cosmos*.

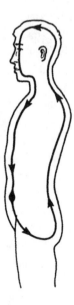

*Fig. 8.2 Small Universal Chi Flow*

When a person has attained the *Small Universal Chi Flow*, his energy supply is never-ending. As he uses his energy for various purposes, he replenishes it from the universe. However, Small Universal Chi Kung is not easy to do, and it takes time to develop. For many sportsmen, mastering *Abdominal Breathing* is quite sufficient for their energy needs.

### Breathe Better, Think More Clearly

Many experiments using Western scientific principles and instruments have been carried out recently in China to test, and subsequently verify, the traditional claims made by Chi Kung masters through the ages, such as that Chi Kung enhances one's stamina, endurance, reflexes, and judgment. As these tests are too numerous and technical to be described here, just two examples are briefly reported below.

The Shanghai Second Tuberculosis Hospital successfully employs Chi Kung therapy as the main—often the sole—means of curing patients, only occasionally prescribing antibiotics to relieve severe symptoms. In a series of experiments in 1965 on patients who had been cured, researchers found that after practicing Chi Kung four times a day for three months, the movements of their diaphragms during breathing increased from an average of 1.8 mm to 5.88 mm; their breathing rates dropped from an average of 19.5 to 15 times a minute; and their lung capacity increased from an average of 428.5 cc to 561.8 cc.

Their improvement during actual Chi Kung practice was striking. Just before their practice, their breathing rates averaged 15.3 times a minute, and their lung capacity 516.5 cc; during practice their breathing rate dropped to only 5.6 times a minute, and their lung capacity increased to 1167.8 cc.[6]

In another series of experiments carried out by the Neuroscience Department of the Shanghai First Medical College in 1962 on healthy participants, researchers found that when the participants closed their eyes in a calm situation, both the experimental group and the control group registered brain wave frequencies of 9–11 times a second (the alpha level). When they opened their eyes, frequency moved to the beta level (14–25 times a second).

When the experimental group started doing Chi Kung, their brain wave frequency returned first to the alpha level, then moved to between six and seven times a second—the theta level—while the control group, who did not perform Chi Kung, continued at the beta level. The members of the experimental group were fully aware of events around them while they were involved in their Chi Kung exercises. As all the participants were healthy, the theta level of the experimental group suggests that Chi Kung enables practitioners to be calm yet alert.[7]

### Basic Ingredients for Champions

Because of poor breathing habits, most people use less than a third of their lung capacity. The air sacs (alveoli) in the other two-thirds of the lungs have become lazy through lack of use. Even with the active air sacs, many of them and their tubes (bronchi) are choked with pollutants.

We use the best breathing methods in Chi Kung. By keeping our breathing deep and slow, we gradually cleanse our active air sacs of pollutants. Deep breathing enables more oxygen to reach deeper into the lungs, replacing stale air that has been collected there for a long time by shallow breathers. Gradually more and more passive air sacs are brought to active service, as you can see in *figure 8.3*.

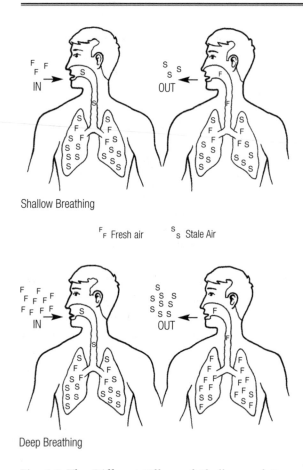

Shallow Breathing

$^F_F$ Fresh air    $^s_s$ Stale Air

Deep Breathing

*Fig. 8.3 The Different Effects of Shallow and Deep Breathing*

Hence Chi Kung enhances the lung capacity, increasing the intake of air from an average of 500 cc per breath to about 1500 cc. Chi Kung masters even achieve a lung capacity of 3000 cc per breath! Moreover, Chi Kung enables a better exchange of oxygen and carbon dioxide. All this means that Chi Kung exponents have a better supply of energy.

Our bodies are well provided with capillaries, which are collateral or sub-branches of meridians called *luo* in Chinese. In one square centimeter on the skin, there are about thirty capillaries, but only two or three are filled with blood in an average person. In a Chi Kung exponent, as many as ten to fifteen are filled with blood. This is what is meant by the expression, "Chi Kung cleanses the meridians and promotes chi and blood circulation." This does not cause a greater loss of blood if we cut ourselves. Chi Kung practice enhances our natural functioning so that the body will trigger the appropriate mechanism to stop the bleeding.

Translated into everyday terms, this means better blood circulation to bring warmth and nutrients to all our cells. Equally important, though less noticeable, is a more efficient disposal system for cleansing our bodies of waste products and dead cells. Each time we breathe out, millions of dead cells are disposed of; each time we breathe in, millions of new cells are born. Indeed, there is more than poetry in the saying that breathing is the very foundation of life, and Chi Kung is, among other things, the art of correct breathing. In this way, Chi Kung enhances our self-regenerative system.

An average person breathes about sixteen times a minute. A Chi Kung practitioner breathes only about five or six times a minutes, as his breathing has become slow and deep through practice. Slow, deep breathing not only provides a better and smoother supply of energy, it is also directly related to mental freshness and tranquility. The slower and deeper the breathing, the calmer a person is, and the less likely he is to become breathless or fatigued.

Chi Kung slows down a person's brain wave frequency, from more than fifteen times a second to around ten times a second, thus enabling him to stay at the alpha level even during normal situations. This explains why Chi Kung masters are always calm, even when faced with demanding situations. It also enables them to develop sound judgment and instant reflexes, as well as to make quick decisions.

It was for these wonderful benefits—health and fitness, a more abundant and efficient energy supply, faster recovery from injury, better stamina and endurance, the freshness of mind to make and carry out quick decisions, and tranquility at all times—that kungfu masters in the past used Chi Kung to enhance their fighting skills. If it worked for kungfu masters—whose stamina and endurance had to last during long hours of fighting, and for whom the wrong decision or slow action could cost them their lives—it can work for modern sportsmen who want to be champions.

### A Suggested Program for Sportsmen

Many Chi Kung students practice their techniques exactly as prescribed by their instructors for fear that faulty practice might lead to serious side effects. While there is truth in this, one need not be unduly worried. Unless you deliberately force yourself to the limit, Chi Kung exercises are generally safer than most forms of sports training. And if you understand the underlying principles, which are abundantly explained in this book, you can choose and even modify the exercises to suit your particular needs. The following is a program that will suit most sportsmen (and sportswomen).

Every morning spend about five minutes practicing *Lifting The Sky* and *Carrying The Moon.* Then follow this with another five minutes of *Induced Chi Flow,* which will cleanse you of any internal injuries which you may unwittingly sustain. End with five minutes of *Standing Meditation,* where you feel yourself at peace with the whole of the cosmos.

Every evening or night, start with *Lifting The Sky,* doing it about ten times. Then practice *Abdominal Breathing* for about eight minutes. End with *Standing Meditation* for about five minutes, during which time once or twice visualize yourself performing those perfect moves or techniques that will make you a champion.

About fifteen minutes per session is quite sufficient, but you must be regular and consistent in your training; practicing off and on will not bring much benefit. If you cannot practice twice a day, then do so at least once, alternating the procedures each day.

You will probably be surprised at your improvement after three months of daily practice. If you make this program part of your training, you will be rewarded with the ingredients that make a champion—abundant energy, quick decision-making, and sound judgment.

### Increasing Stamina and Endurance

Cheng is an amateur long-distance runner. He can run 1 km with just one breath, and after running 20 km he looks as if he has just taken a leisurely walk! How does he do it? One effective method is the *Art of a Thousand Steps,* a technique practiced in the past by the kungfu disciples of the Shaolin Monastery.

First you must be able to do *Abdominal Breathing.* If you cannot do this well, you should turn back to Chapter 4 and start practicing. Use *Abdominal Breathing* throughout this exercise. Of course you must also be properly dressed, including wearing suitable shoes for running long distances.

Do *Abdominal Breathing* three times. Then as you breathe in through your nose for the fourth time, start running on the spot. After taking a full breath into the abdomen, hold your breath gently for about six counts as you run. Your mouth should be slightly open so that some breath may escape. Then breathe slowly and gently into your abdomen, while continuing to run on the spot.

You will still have some breath in your abdomen when you start to breathe in again. It is very important that you always keep this reserve of energy in your abdomen; it must never be less than thirty percent of the energy you breathe in. If you have difficulty keeping this reserve of energy, it means that you have not done the preliminary *Abdominal Breathing* exercise properly.

Continue breathing and holding your breath while running on the spot. Note that you should not stop running, and there should be no conscious effort to breathe out. After running on the spot for about five minutes, walk about for one or two minutes. Maintain your *Abdominal Breathing*, but stop holding your breath. This completes the first stage of the exercise.

You should not be panting after the exercise; if you are, you probably have not performed the breathing and holding properly. Practice this stage for about two weeks, gradually increasing the length of time you hold your breath, as well as the length of the exercise. But you must not hold your breath for so long that you have less than thirty percent reserve energy, and you must not continue the exercise for so long that you end it panting.

Proceed to the second stage only when you are totally proficient at stage one. In this stage, follow the same procedure but towards the end, run about thirty steps instead of staying on the spot. End the exercise with walking and *Abdominal Breathing* as before. Later you may not have to count while holding your breath.

Continue practicing, but each day, or every alternate day, run a few more actual steps instead of staying on the spot. Eventually you should not be running on the spot at all, but start your actual running immediately after the initial *Abdominal Breathing*. But you must still complete the exercise without feeling breathless.

In stage three, continue adding more steps gradually until you can run the basic one thousand steps without panting for breath. Then you will easily be able to run long distances. As with all other Chi Kung exercises, the essential factor is consistent, regular practice. You must practice at least once a day until you have the skill and energy to run the basic thousand steps.

The crucial thing is to breathe in gently, hold your breath as you run until you have used up about seventy percent of your energy, then breathe in to replenish it. At all times you must have thirty percent reserve energy.

We can apply this technique to other sports and games. Whether in football, martial arts, or any other vigorous activity, if you can maintain your rate of slow, deep breathing despite fast movements, you will find that you have a lot of stamina and endurance.

# CHAPTER NINE

# Enhancing Sexual Performance

> Many human beings, in fact all too many, seem to think that our sexual apparatus consists largely of the genitals and associated structures. They are wrong. The sexual apparatus consists of the entire human body, most of the essentials of which are not only necessary for the arousal of sex desire and the attainment of orgasm, but are also intimately involved in climactic release.
>
> Dr. Albert Ellis, *The Art and Science of Love*

### Sex, Instinct and Spirituality

What is the common factor in all these arts: the *Technique of Changing Energy to Essence*, the *Art of Strengthening the Kidneys*, the *Art of Retaining Gold*, the *Art of Returning to Spring*, the *Technique of Raising Yang*, the *Inside-Room Technique*, and the *Art of Vitality*? They are all Chi Kung arts, and they are all concerned with teaching practitioners, especially male practitioners, how to get more out of sex.

Confucius said, "Satisfying hunger for food, and hunger for sex are basic human instincts." But the great sage and other masters warned that one must not abuse sex, and certainly not indulge in it licentiously.

Some Eastern cultures regard sex as sacred, even as a means to spirituality. Wall sculptures of gods and goddesses in ecstatic embraces are quite common in Indian temple buildings. Statues of deities in sexual poses may be found behind the screens of some Tibetan temples.

How does sex lead to spirituality? One theory suggests that the intense emotion of erotic love approximates the wonders of the deep religious experience. Another suggests that the universe is a spiritual unity of the male and female principles, and the copulation of man and woman manifests this cosmic union. A third theory, believed by some Taoist sects, claims that man draws feminine energy from a woman to unite with his masculine energy, or vice versa, to promote cosmic *yin-yang* harmony for achieving immortality.

### An Erotic Path to Immortality?

However, the records of great masters who attained high levels of spirituality show that the joy of deep religious experience is distinctly different from sexual excitement. In deep levels of meditation, great masters of different religious and philosophical beliefs have independently, but unanimously, found the cosmos to be an undifferentiated unity. There has never been any record of Taoist masters attaining sainthood or immortality through sexual intercourse.

This, however, does not necessarily imply that sex is detrimental to spiritual development. Seducing students on the pretext of injecting them with power, or asking them to desert their families so as to serve so-called masters, is certainly unscrupulous and wrong. On the other hand, employing Chi Kung or other techniques to enhance sexual performance for sincere purposes is wholesome and wise.

Of the various philosophical schools of Chi Kung, the Taoist is the richest in techniques for sex. In fact, as I have said, some Taoist sects even employ sex as a means to spiritual development, though many Taoist masters regard this as a deviant practice resulting from shallow knowledge, or as exploiting the ignorance of others for selfish lust.

Some Taoist students believe that there are three approaches to immortality, namely heaven, earth, and human. In the heaven approach, immortality may be attained through the heavenly breath, that is, by uniting with the cosmos through Chi Kung practice. In the earth approach, one may become a saint by eating a pearl of elixir prepared through alchemy. In the human approach, one may attain spirituality by merging the male and female principles through sexual intercourse.

Many Taoist masters say that the earth and human approaches are debased, adulterated forms that resulted from an inadequate understanding of arcane Taoist teachings which are often written in symbolic language. An example of a mistaken interpretation of the earth approach—the golden pearl of energy—was given in Chapter 3.

### A Saint Immersed in a Rainbow Stream

Similarly, reading an arcane text which is written in a romantic language, without knowing its secret meaning, may lead uninformed students to interpret it incorrectly. The following verse is taken from a very important Taoist classic, *The Realizing of Truth*, written by Zhang Bo Duan in the eleventh century.

> If you want to be a saint, be a heavenly saint.
> Only the golden pearl will provide the extreme.
> When two unite, and blissful feelings merge,
> They become tigress and dragon in ecstatic scream.
> Wu Ji the match-maker has successfully blessed
> The husband and wife locked in a happy dream.
> Their effort achieved, they face the palace gate
> And ascend to heaven immersed in a rainbow stream.

Colloquially, to be a saint may mean to have an ecstatic sexual experience, and ascending to heaven reinforces this blissful feeling. The dragon and the tigress represent the male and female principles. It is easy for the romantically inclined to interpret this verse as attaining spirituality through blissful love-making.

But what do the experts say about it? There are five levels of sainthood, and to be a heavenly saint is to attain the highest level. The golden pearl is the accumulation of cosmic energy at the abdomen. "Two," in "when two unite," refers to the *kan* trigram and the *li* trigram of the Eight Trigram formation. *Kan* symbolizes water, and refers to man's original essence, whereas *li* symbolizes fire, and refers to man's original spirit. "When two unite," is an arcane expression for a developmental stage in Chi Kung practice when the practitioner transforms his essence into energy. The next line about the dragon and the tigress refers to an act of will to merge man's post-natal essence and spirit.

*Wu* and *ji* are two of the Chinese "ten heavenly stems," and refer to the earth process in the concept of the *Five Elemental Processes*, symbolizing willpower. Willpower is needed to combine essence with spirit in Chi Kung practice, hence *wu ji* is sometimes nicknamed "yellow woman," the matchmaker. Essence and spirit, two of the three inner aspects of man (the other aspect is energy), are further symbolized by the wife and the husband respectively. When essence and spirit are well merged, the practitioner is calm and happy. When he is successful in his efforts, the Taoist faces the prospect of becoming a saint and ascending to heaven in all his glory.

In short, the verse is a concise and concealed description of a Chi Kung technique to attain sainthood. The adept, using willpower to harmonize his energy flow merges his physical with his spiritual body to achieve immortality.

### Sexual Endurance and Multiple Performance

Besides such arcane writings, which purposely mislead the uninitiated into believing them to be amorous descriptions, Taoist texts are also rich in real—and explicit—advice concerning sex. The *Inner Classic of Bao Puz Zi* unambiguously advises:

> Man should not abstain from sexual intercourse until he becomes sick. However, if he unreservedly follows his desires, he only shortens his life. But those who know the art—that is, those who ride on horses and yet can nourish their brains, return the essence to nourish their bodies, extract jade juices from golden ponds, abstain from sexual activities when environmental or psychological circumstances are unfavorable—those who know all these techniques for use inside the room, can still be handsome even when they age, and be able to live their potential life span.

"Riding on horses" does not refer to positions for sexual intercourse. It means bringing the golden pearl of energy round the body in a *Small Universal Chi Flow*—like a horse on a racecourse—so that this energy will flow to the head and nourish the mental faculties. By an act of will—and a lot of practice—this circuit of energy flow round the body is performed during the sex act. This will prevent ejaculation, thus increasing sexual endurance. Endurance here, of course, means the ability to perform and enjoy the experience for longer; it does not imply any hardship during intercourse.

If you can "return essence to nourish yourself," you can, whether you are a man or a woman, not only prolong intercourse, but also have sex several times without draining yourself. Essence refers to a man's sperm or a woman's egg and vaginal juices.

This technique was taught to emperors in the past to help them enjoy multiple performances. Basically, it consists in withholding ejaculation yet savoring carnal delights.

Records suggest that exponents of this technique initially missed some of the intense enjoyment of sex, but as they became proficient at it their enjoyment became greater than in normal intercourse. We have little evidence to support or refute this claim because we discourage the use of this technique as it is likely to be abused. Nevertheless, there is nothing wrong in using it with sincere intent.

### Jade Juices from Golden Ponds

Some Taoist priests had several wives. Although some of these priests were over sixty years old, their complexions were often rosy, their eyes sparkling, and their voices "rich like resonant bells." Their secret was "extracting jade juices from golden ponds."

One concept, known as *Inside-Room Art*, concerns methods for extracting jade juices (a collective name for vaginal secretions and feminine energy), as well as detailed descriptions of erogenous zones, foreplay techniques, the right timing, and erotic movements. The following is an abridged version of a lengthy description of the build-up to the extraction of jade juices, taken from *The Taoist Secret Art of Immortality:*

The foreplay should take into consideration the network of energy flow. Caresses, therefore, start from the body's extremities and move to the center. Where is the center? The genitals, of course....

The proper place to start is the woman's middle finger. Place her palm on your palm, and using your thumb, gently caress first her middle finger, then her index and fourth fingers....

Stroking the arm is different from caressing the fingers. The inside of the elbow is well embedded with chi. If you stroke this part properly, her yang chi will rise to her shoulders, move down her bosom and hips, then to her genitals. Here, do not use your thumb, but use your other four fingers....

Place your nose on her neck to nudge her. Why do you not use your mouth? Because your nose can emit breath that will stimulate her chi beneath her skin....

Place your mouth on her throat and nibble fairly hard....Then place your mouth on her bosom to suck at her nipple....First place your lips over the whole of her nipple. Let your mouth warm the base of her nipple for some time before you start to use your tongue to lick the tip of her nipple. If you lick at the nipple too early, you may cause too much excitement, which may result in negative chi arising....

Ultimately, after he has aroused her to ecstasy, causing her *chi* to focus at her vagina, the man draws jade juices from the woman, through his penis, into his body. This "extraction of jade juices from golden ponds" will make him fit and healthy, even in old age, but will literally drain the poor woman dry.

This, of course, is highly immoral. We believe that no one should derive benefits, no matter how great or tempting, from the suffering of others. Taoist masters tell us that such unethical sexual practices, like black magic and superstitious rituals, are corrupt deviations by people who do not understand the true meaning of Taoism. Any practice that willfully harms any other being just cannot be right.

### Appreciating Sexual Experience

Sex is a wholesome experience that God (or Buddha, or Allah, or the Tao) wants us to enjoy. If we want to improve our performance so that we can better appreciate sex, there are effective methods we can use which do not involve hurting others. *Submerged Breathing* is one such method.

It has helped to cure Teng, a millionaire in his sixties, of his sexual impotency. It has also rejuvenated Ricky, a retired government officer in his fifties.

"Sifu," he said over the phone. "I have a problem. Practically every day for the past week, I have made love to my wife."

"Did you enjoy it?" I asked, rather foolishly.

"Tremendously."

"Did you feel worn out or unwell after making love?"

"No! In fact, I feel fresh and energetic, more so than in my younger days. It was never like this before. But my wife is worried. She thinks something must have gone wrong."

"Don't worry, you're perfectly all right. You're reaping the benefits of Submerged Breathing!"

### A Small Wheel to Improve Performance

*Submerged Breathing* is based on *Abdominal Breathing* (see Chapter 6).

1.  Stand upright and relaxed with your feet fairly close together. Place both palms on your *qihai*, the *dan tian* (energy field) about two inches below the navel.
2.  Deflate your abdomen and breathe out your negative energy.
3.  Breathe cosmic energy through your nose into your abdomen. Your abdomen will of course rise as you breathe in. Pause for a second or two.

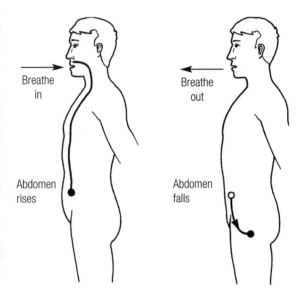

*Fig. 9.1 Submerged Breathing*

energy flow in your body may not follow the instruction of your mind. This is natural. It takes some time (generally ranging from two weeks to two months of daily training) before you can effectively use your mind to direct the energy flow. If you persist in your training, however, you will soon find that you can actually direct it with your mind.

After performing *Submerged Breathing* about thirty-six times, drop your hands to your sides. Close your eyes (if you have not unconsciously done so earlier) and experience the tranquility of *Standing Meditation* for a short time (which can be from a few seconds to one or two minutes). Then place your mind in the area of your kidneys. Do not ask how you can do it; just do it. Do not exert any force: like all other visualization exercises, it must be done gently.

You may experience a feeling of warmth around the kidneys after some time. Visualize a flow of energy from your back at your kidneys to

4. Deflate your abdomen and breathe out through your mouth, but visualize cosmic energy (presently in your *qihai* vital point) gently flowing down to your *huiyin* vital point, the *dan tian* just before the anus. Pause for a second or two.
5. Breathe cosmic energy into your abdomen. Pause.
6. Breathe out, visualizing energy flowing down to your *huiyin*.

Repeat this process of breathing into your abdomen, and breathing out with energy flowing to your *huiyin* about thirty-six times. (When you start, do it about ten times, and gradually increase to thirty-six as you progress.) Cosmic energy flows from the universe into your *qihai* as you breathe in, and flows from your *qihai* to your *huiyin* as you breathe out.

Initially when you breathe out, you may feel that energy is actually flowing up to your mouth, despite visualizing it flowing down to your anus. In other words, at the initial stage, the actual

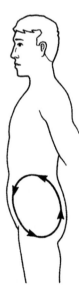

*Fig. 9.2 Wheel of Energy Flow for Erotic Delights*

your front at your navel, then down to your genitals, and up again to the base of your spine, and back to your kidneys, in a continuous small wheel of energy flow. Enjoy it for about ten minutes. But it is important that your visualization should be done *very gently*.

To complete this exercise, think of your kidneys. Rub your palms together until they are warm, and place them on your kidneys. Then rub them again, and place them on your eyes as you open them.

Massage your face gently and walk about briskly.

Chi Kung experts are noted for their tremendous sexual prowess. If you practice this Chi Kung exercise conscientiously, you will probably understand why. But never abuse it. The vitality we get from this and other exercises is intended to make life meaningful and satisfying for ourselves and for others; if we use it extravagantly or licentiously, we will harm ourselves.

# CHAPTER TEN

# Chi Kung and Women's Sexuality

Whether women are better than men I cannot say—but I can say they are certainly no worse.

Golda Meir

### An Unmistakable Case of Rejuvenation

Men and women are not born equal—and the difference goes far beyond their sexual organs. There are many things that women can do better than men. Of course there are also other things—like carrying heavy luggage—that men generally do better.

One significant difference between the sexes is that women undergo menopause, while men do not. Many women suffer at this time because menopause not only disturbs their hormonal balance, but may also make them feel that they are losing their sexual appeal. Fortunately, practicing Chi Kung is an efficient remedy for both these problems.

For many years, Mrs. Leong, who was in her fifties, had to go to a special hospital for two or three weeks each year because of a problem with her colon. But the hospital could only alleviate her symptoms, not cure her. Finally she turned to Chi Kung as an alternative. She practiced conscientiously, and after about nine months she achieved the breakthrough of the *Small Universe*—she could channel her energy round her body smoothly along her *ren* and *du* meridians. By then her problem with her colon had disappeared.

Mrs. Leong progressed to practice the *Big Universe* Chi Kung, which aims to channel energy through the twelve primary meridians. In the middle of this program, a remarkable thing happened. She started to menstruate again—ten years after her menopause! She was worried, but a thorough medical examination confirmed that it was not cancerous bleeding, but menstruation. When she consulted a Chinese physician for a second opinion, he congratulated her on her rejuvenation. She now looks and feels ten years younger.

She persuaded her husband, who did not believe in Chi Kung until it saved him his wife's hospital fees, to practice the art. Later, he confided that he was glad he had taken it up as it gave him the vitality he needed to enjoy his wife's renewed sexuality.

### Warming the Womb for Fertility

Chi Kung gave Nancy, a young woman of twenty-six, a different, but related, benefit. She had no children, though she and her husband longed for some, and tried hard to have them. Twice Nancy conceived but then miscarried. Medical examinations showed the fetuses to have been normal. Nancy told me that all the conventional doctors she had consulted insisted that she was healthy and normal; but all her Chinese physicians said that she was sick and that her kidneys were weak.

According to Chinese medical philosophy, illness can be classified into two groups: "solid" diseases, where the causes are readily visible, like a bacterial infection or a structural defect; and "empty" diseases, where the causes are "invisible," such as a blockage of energy flow or a functional disorder.

If you feel sick, but your doctor cannot find the cause, you should start questioning whether yours is an empty sickness. "Empty" here is, of course, a figurative term; it suggests that the illness is apparently empty of causes. Empty diseases, because they are insidious, can often be more serious than solid ones. Practicing Chi Kung is an excellent way to cure them. However, if the disease is solid, conventional medicine is quicker.

Nancy's illness was empty; her womb was too "cold" to be capable of holding a fetus. The logical remedy was to "warm" the womb. In more conventional Western terms, Nancy's womb did not function properly, probably because of some nervous or hormonal disorder.

To help her "warm" her womb, I taught Nancy *Lifting The Sky, Carrying The Moon*, and *Nourishing The Kidneys* (see below). These *dao yin* movements led to *Induced Chi Flow*, whereby Nancy allowed vital energy to flow spontaneously inside her body. This cleansed her meridians (enabling the smooth flow of electric impulses along her nerves, hence enhancing her feedback system) and restored her *yin-yang* harmony (correcting hormonal imbalance). Finally she remained still in her *Standing Meditation* and visualized *chi* focusing at her kidneys, thereby generating vital energy at those organs which Chinese medical thinking maintains are directly related to sexual performance.

After about six months, Nancy conceived, and when their healthy baby boy arrived, she and her husband were overjoyed.

### Nourishing The Kidneys for Vitality

In Chinese medical philosophy, the kidneys are directly related to male virility and female fertility. Almost all sexual disorders are connected with the kidney system.

Even if you do not want sexual virility or fertility, *Nourishing The Kidneys* is still very beneficial as it gives you overall vitality and health. Moreover this exercise can help your hair grow, bringing hope to balding men.

Stand with your feet fairly close together. Think of the *yongquan* vital points, situated at the soles of your feet, for a few seconds.

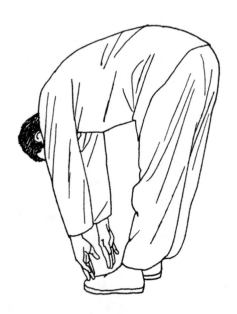

*Fig. 10.1 Touching the Toes*

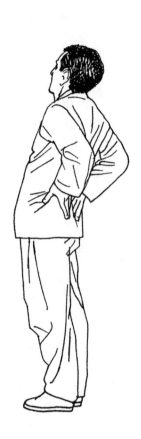

Fig. 10.2 Nourishing the Kidneys

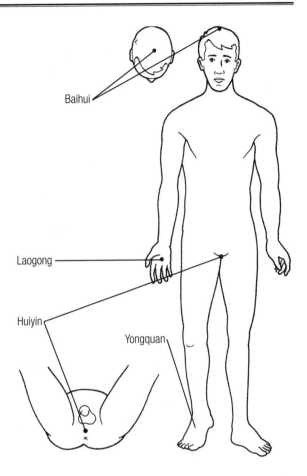

Fig. 10.2 Nourishing the Kidneys

Then, with your knees straight, bend down so that you touch your toes with your fingers, breathing out gently at the same time, as in *figure 10.1*. Simultaneously visualize *chi* flowing along your spine from your *huiyin* (the vital point near the anus) to your *baihui* (the vital point at the crown of your head.)

Pause in this position for about two seconds and visualize your *chi* at your *laogong* vital points, which are situated at the center of your palms. If your aim is to prevent baldness, focus your *chi* at your *baihui* instead of your *laogong*.

Next raise your body and gently breathe in,

visualizing your palms charged with cosmic energy. Then place both palms at your back at your kidneys, slightly arching your back, as in *figure 10.2*. Breathe out slowly with a sizzling sound, with your teeth close together. At the same time visualize *chi* from your palms flowing into your kidneys, massaging and nourishing them. Next, visualize vital energy flowing from your kidneys to your bladder and sex organs.

Then straighten your body and drop your arms at your sides to return to the starting position. Think of your *yongquan* vital points again.

The aim of this exercise is not just to stretch your leg muscles, though you will get this benefit as a bonus. The main purpose is to cleanse the kidney and urinary bladder meridian systems and to strengthen the kidneys themselves, not just to provide a better blood filter (though this is a very important function too) but also to enhance your sexual responses and pleasures.

This exercise, especially in conjunction with other relevant Chi Kung exercises such as the combination I taught Nancy, has helped many men to regain their potency, and many women who had previously been considered barren to bear children.

### Absorbing the Moon's Essence

In traditional Chinese society, not being able to bear children was considered a cardinal sin, and an excuse for the husband to find another wife. While this attitude is dying out, not being able to have children when you want them can be extremely distressing. The above Chi Kung exercises may bring hope to childless couples, as it has done to many of my students.

Another interesting Chi Kung exercise was prescribed by an imperial professor of medicine, Chao Yuan Fang, for infertile women.

Just as the moon rises and the sun goes down, stand facing the moon. Hold your breath for eight counts. Then tilt your head backward and slowly and deeply draw in the moon's essence. When this *yin* energy of the moon is abundant, it will clear the pathways connected with childbirth, as well as nourishing the brain, so that even women over forty-nine years of age can continue to have children and those who have been barren for some time will find their fertility restored. If you practice consistently and conscientiously, you will also achieve longevity.

This technique is certainly exotic, but if you are tempted to laugh at it as outlandish, remember that Chao Yuan Fang was one of the greatest physicians China has produced, and many of his Chi Kung techniques and medical principles have so far been found correct and useful. Perhaps our modern scientists should investigate the hypothesis that energy from the moon can increase our sexual fertility.

### Nurturing the Fetus

Chi Kung not only increases the chances of conception, but also nurtures the fetus during its development in the womb. Practically all my female students who conceived while they were practicing Chi Kung, and the male students who continued practicing Chi Kung while their wives were pregnant, told me that their babies were more healthy, energetic and intelligent than others.

I do not encourage expectant mothers to practice Chi Kung during pregnancy—though it is actually good for them if they do it correctly—because I do not want them to run the risk, no matter how small it may be, of harming the fetus through wrong practice. But if expectant mothers who are already Chi Kung practitioners feel confident and proficient enough not to make any serious mistakes in their practice, they can do gentle Chi Kung exercises like *Abdominal Breathing* (without pressing the abdomen with the palms) and visualization. Ordinary breathing can also be used in place of *Abdominal Breathing*. But exercises that involve stretching or vigorous movements, like most *dao yin* exercises and *Induced Chi Flow*, are not suitable.

Breathe in gently and think of good cosmic energy flowing in and nurturing the fetus. Then stand, sit, or lie down comfortably, and gently visualize the fetus developing into a lovely, healthy baby who will eventually be delivered pleasantly in a natural way. All these must be done gently, very gently.

There are other ways to nurture the fetus. If the expectant mother is within the good energy field created by Chi Kung exponents practicing in a group, the cosmic energy radiated will be beneficial to the fetus. But she should avoid sick people practicing Chi Kung for therapy because the negative energy radiated could be harmful.

If a healthy father is in a meditative Chi Kung state and thinks of his baby, he can generate good energy to benefit his baby while it is in the mother's womb if the mother is nearby. This sounds bizarre to the uninitiated, but like many other exotic techniques in Chi Kung, it can be explained quite logically.

Another way is to channel *chi* directly to the fetus, but this must be done by a competent master. In some ways it is similar to the blessing of the fetus by a spiritual teacher.

### Small is Beautiful

Frequent childbirth may cause a problem that many women dread but do not like discussing with others—the weakening of the vaginal muscles, resulting in an enlarged vagina. As a comprehensive art, Chi Kung can help here too. The following exercise will alleviate this problem, and you do not have to have borne children to enjoy the benefits. So long as you believe that small is beautiful, you (and your partner) will find the effort spent practicing it well worth while.

This art was practiced by Zhao Fei Yan, one of the great beauties in Chinese history who was renowned for her small size. She was as amorous

as she was beautiful, and had numerous affairs, although she remained unmarried. But when the Emperor took her as one of his concubines, he found her vagina so tight that he thought she was a virgin. What was her secret? "The Art of Lifting the Anus," she said.

Stand upright and relaxed, with feet fairly close together. By an act of will, lift up your anus as if you were holding back your bowel motion. Breathe in as you do so. Hold your breath and your position for a short while—from two seconds to a minute, depending on your comfort.

Then relax and breathe out *gently*. Continually breathing out with too much force may result in a prolapsed rectum or varicose veins, or in the case of men, a hernia. But do not worry too much about this happening; you will receive sufficient warning in the form of pain or discomfort, and if you heed the warning and correct your method, you will be all right.

Repeat the lifting and relaxing of your anus as often as you feel comfortable. A rough guide for beginners is thirty times. Practice daily in the morning and in the evening or at night. Gradually increase the frequency to three hundred times, and later to five hundred.

You can also perform the exercise lying down, and it is an important technique in many other Chi Kung exercises. Unlike the other exercises in this book, however, I have no case histories to prove that it works. I could not ask my female students the size of their vagina, nor are any of them likely to come to me and say, "Sifu, my vagina has become smaller!" So, for the validity of this exercise, you will have to trust the evidence of Lady Zhao, as well as the records of other Chi Kung authorities.

# CHAPTER ELEVEN

# Acquiring a Blooming Face and a Shapely Figure

*Wanting to be beautiful is a woman's instinct.*
*Chinese proverb*

## Acquiring a Childlike Complexion

Chi Kung not only makes you healthy, it can also be used as a beauty aid. We shall start with the skin, since it covers some 20,000 square centimeters in an average adult and is therefore the first thing people notice about us. If you give some time and effort to Chi Kung, it will reward you with a blooming, childlike complexion.

Some of the defects that mar the beauty of our skin are acne, pimples, rashes, wrinkles, dryness and oiliness. The cause of these blemishes is that the skin fails to function properly; there is over- or under-production of oils, and inadequate blood circulation to clear waste products and to bring nourishment to the skin tissues. The failure of the endocrine glands to produce the right proportions of hormones can also affect the skin.

Hence, keeping skin healthy and beautiful requires not just localized treatment, but a holistic approach, covering the whole body. Covering the skin with cream or powder merely hides skin defects. It is better to remove these defects, and then to use cosmetics, if needed, to enhance, rather than hide, the skin.

When we practice Chi Kung, *chi* or vital energy flows at five progressive levels: skin, flesh, meridians, bones, and internal organs. Thus, the skin is among the first to show the benefits of Chi Kung practice. A universal effect of Chi Kung practice on my students is that after a few months they feel warm and their skin looks fresh and lively. This is because when *chi* flows along the skin, it promotes better blood circulation, which cleanses the skin of waste products and brings vitality to its tissues.

Acne, pimples, and rashes, however, will take a little longer to clear. When the flow of *chi* has harmonized the hormonal production of the sebaceous and other glands in the skin, these surface blemishes will disappear. Long-standing skin problems like scaly skin and wrinkles will take still longer, as they are related to other aspects of our body.

As you continue practicing, Chi Kung will cleanse your body of toxic waste. For a short while, your breath may become heavier and your body smell stronger and you may pass off gases more frequently than before. These are some of the ways your body clears itself of waste products. But do not worry; soon you will not only look sweet but also smell nice.

Almost any Chi Kung exercises will produce these benefits. *Dao yin* and *Induced Chi Flow* are particularly useful, and *Lifting The Sky* is an excellent exercise as it engenders the flow of chi over the body.

### Massage for a Blooming Face

Perform *Lifting The Sky* about twenty times, thinking of vital energy shimmering under your skin after each exercise as you pause to appreciate the tingling effect of the *chi* flow. Do not be surprised if you feel as if there are insects crawling over your body. This is the effect of *chi* flowing in your skin.

If your body sways or moves about after this series of *Lifting The Sky*, enjoy the *Induced Chi Flow* for about five minutes. Then proceed to *Standing Meditation* for another five minutes. If there is no swaying, skip the *Induced Chi Flow* and proceed to *Standing Meditation*. Complete the program with Chi Kung face massage, as explained below.

Massaging or stimulating energy points is an important part of Chi Kung therapy. Unlike *Induced Chi Flow* which is generally holistic, massaging energy points is a thematic approach, employing specific points for particular diseases.

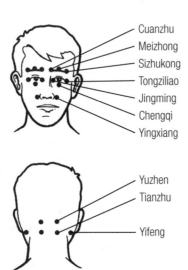

*Fig. 11.1 Some Energy Points for Face Massage*

This technique is closely related to massage therapy, and similar to acupuncture, which, along with Chi Kung therapy, herbalism, and surgery, are major branches of Chinese medicine. See *figure 11.1* for the relevant energy points.

1. Use your index or middle fingers to massage the *jingming* energy points located at the inner lower corners of your eyes a few times. The idea is to stimulate energy to flow.
2. Then massage the *cuanzhu* energy points found at the inner ends of the eyebrows. Stroke the entire eyebrows a few times with your fingers, moving from the inside out.
3. Then massage the *meizhong* energy points.
4. Move along the eyebrows to the outer ends and massage the *sizhukong* energy points.
5. Next massage the *tongziliao* energy points, then the *chengqi* energy points, and return to the *jingming* energy points, thus making a complete cycle round the eyes.
6. Use the thumb and the middle or index finger to stroke the ridge of the nose from the top near the eyebrows downwards to its base a few times.
7. Then massage the *yingxiang* energy points.
8. Place your thumbs at the hollows behind the ears where you can feel the pulse at the neck, and massage the *yifeng* energy points.
9. Then use the broad bases of your thumbs (not the thumbs or fingers) to massage the *taiyang* energy points at the temples.
10. Next, using two or three fingers together and starting from the inner, lower corners, massage the rims round your eyes, starting with small circles, and making them bigger and bigger until you are massaging the whole face, then move up the head from front to back, and down the neck.
11. Finally, place both hands at the back of your neck so that the fingers are almost touching each other, and cup your ears with both

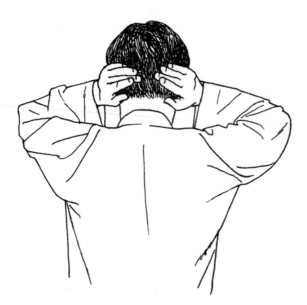

*Fig. 11.2 Sounding the Heavenly Drum*

palms, as in *figure 11.2*. Place your index fingers on your middle fingers, and using the middle fingers as pivots, flick your index fingers down on to the back of your head, gently hitting the *yuzhen* and *tianzhu* energy points twenty-four times. Your ears should be firmly covered by your palms, and you will hear a sonorous "droom…droom" sound, described as *Sounding the Heavenly Drum*. This massage will give you a blooming face and sparkling eyes.

### Treat the Cause, Not the Symptom

With a blooming face, sparkling eyes, and a glowing complexion, the next step is to acquire a shapely figure. The Chi Kung approach to slimming is different from that of the West. From the Chi Kung perspective, vigorous exercises like aerobics and running are not recommended because they are too demanding; they waste a lot

of energy, and the practitioners may become flabby or even unwell once they stop their vigorous exercises. Chi Kung philosophy contends that forcefully removing extra protein and carbohydrate by aggressive burning of energy is both unnatural and unhealthy.

Dieting as a means of slimming is even worse. Besides denying you the pleasures of eating, dieting deprives the body of the necessary energy for work and play, and weakens various important body systems and functions, with far-reaching consequences.

It is a common misconception that depriving ourselves of food will reduce our mass. In fact, some overweight people eat very little, yet remain overweight; and some thin people eat a lot, yet remain thin. The problem lies with hormonal dysfunction. Overweight people do not produce enough hormones to break down the food they eat into energy, whereas thin people break down their food too much, so that they do not have any excess to build up their mass. In Chinese medical terms, this is a case of *yin-yang* disharmony.

Once the harmony is restored, the right amount of hormones will be produced to convert food into the right amount of flesh or energy. Even the amount of food you eat will be regulated by nature: if food is needed for fuel or building blocks, complex reactions in the body will make you want to eat. If, out of desire rather than need, you eat too much, your body will produce the necessary hormones to rectify this temporary excess. If you keep on eating, chemical reactions in your body will cause a reduction in your appetite.

The body is actually a wonderful cosmos, but all its autonomous systems can function flawlessly only when *chi*, which feeds all its parts with the right information, is flowing harmoniously. Chi Kung ensures and enhances this harmonious flow of *chi*. Hence, by practicing Chi Kung, you can eat your favorite cakes and chocolates, yet still maintain your figure.

Peggy had a figure that bulged at the middle. In fact, without meaning to be rude, she was like a barrel. She would have loved to be slim, but she loved cakes and chocolates more. After six months of daily Chi Kung, she not only has a good figure, but she maintains her weight while still enjoying her cakes and chocolates, and she is healthier and livelier too! She has remolded herself through Chi Kung, internally carving huge chunks from her middle and replacing them at her hips and bust.

Before we examine the Chi Kung exercises that helped Peggy, it is worth explaining the Chinese medical concept of "branch and root," which can be translated as "symptom and cause."

In addition to treating the patient, not the disease, another cardinal principle of Chinese medicine is to "treat the root [or cause] of the illness, not just the branch [or symptom]." Hence, the preferred treatment for diabetes or peptic ulcers, for example, is not just to inject insulin or cut away the affected portion of the stomach— this is treating the symptom; the Chi Kung treatment is to clear energy blockage (restoring the feedback system), and harmonize *yin-yang* (restoring the hormonal balance), so that the body produces its own hormones, as it has always done before, to neutralize the excess sugar and gastric juices—this is treating the cause.

However, there are occasions when it is necessary to treat the symptom first, such as when it is causing severe suffering or is life-threatening, or when preliminary treatment of the symptom would make it easier to treat the cause later on. For example, if the peptic ulcer is causing great pain, the Chi Kung therapist will first stop the pain by pressing the relevant energy points; but he will also realize that relieving the pain is just an ad hoc measure, and that he must ultimately attack the root cause.

In the same way, eating excessively or dieting as a means to add or reduce weight is treating the symptom, not the cause; so is exercising aggressively to burn off excess weight. The root approach, treating the cause, is to harmonize hormone production, and this can be achieved effectively through Chi Kung.

### From Fat to Shapely

In Peggy's case, I first treated the symptom, not because it was severely painful or life-threatening, but because it would speed up the subsequent treatment of the cause. Her program was as follows.

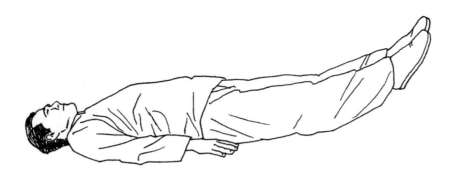

*Fig. 11.3 Drawing the Moon*

Lie flat on your bed or the floor with your arms at your sides. Raise both feet about six inches, and certainly no more than two feet from the floor. Point your toes (see *figure 11.3*).

With your feet together and your knees straight, draw a small circle in the air with your pointed toes. It does not matter whether you move in a clockwise or a counterclockwise direction, but you must move your feet very slowly—not less than half a minute for each circle. If you can continue, draw more circles in the same direction. If not, gently drop your feet and rest for a few seconds. Then repeat the procedure the same number of times in the opposite direction. Remember that you must draw the circle in the air very slowly—it must not take less than half a minute. Rest for a short while and repeat the whole procedure—drawing the circle very slowly the same number of times on both sides.

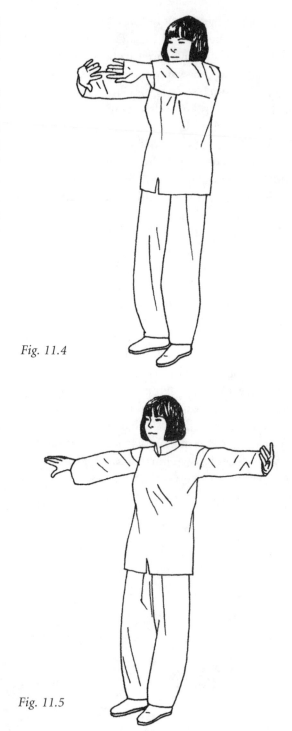

Fig. 11.4

This is called *Drawing The Moon*, and that is all there is to it. Like many of the Chi Kung exercises, the technique is bafflingly simple. The secret, though, is that you *must* practice regularly and consistently, morning and night. A good arrangement is to perform this exercise just before you get up in the morning, and just before you go to sleep at night. There is no taboo associated with it. You may have sex before or after it if you want to. Gradually, as you become more proficient, increase the number of times you draw the circle. By the time you can do ten circles each way, you will have to change your wardrobe!

After *Drawing The Moon* in the morning, get up and perform *Lifting The Sky*. For the night session, you can do *Lifting The Sky* first so that you can go to bed after *Drawing The Moon*. Practice this combination for at least three months, or until your "bulge" has disappeared considerably, before you add the two exercises that follow.

Fig. 11.5

Figs. 11.4-11.5 Separating Water

## Separating Water for a Lovely Bust

Stand with feet fairly close together. Hold both hands in front of you at shoulder level, with your thumbs down, your palms facing forward, and your fingers almost touching, as in *figure 11.4*. Keeping your elbows straight, your arms at shoulders level and your palms at right angles to your wrists, move your arms apart (see *figure 11.5*). At the same time breathe gently and fully through your nose into your chest. Slowly raise your chest as high as you can as you breathe in, and visualize good cosmic energy nourishing and strengthening your bust. Pause for one or two seconds. Then breathe out slowly through your mouth.

Repeat this "separating water" movement about ten times, gradually increasing to about twenty times as you progress. To complete the exercise, after you have moved your arms apart for the last time, without moving your arms turn your palms so that they face downwards, then lower your arms to your sides and simultaneously breathe out through your mouth.

Stand with your feet about shoulder width apart, with your arms hanging loosely at your sides. Rotate your hips about thirty times as if you were using a hula-hoop. You can start in either direction. Then rotate your hips the other way the same number of times.

Next, close your eyes, remain still and think of *chi* circulating round your waist. When you start to move, follow the momentum and enjoy the circular *chi* flow, moving involuntarily. Gently think of your *chi* relocating your flesh at the right places. After about ten minutes, or when you are satisfied, think of your movements coming to a

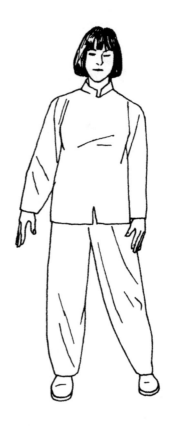

*Fig. 11.6 Circular Chi Flow in Motion*

gentle stop. Complete the exercise with a face massage, as explained on page 73.

If you already have a good figure and want to use these exercises to maintain or enhance it, perform all four exercises: *Lifting The Sky, Drawing The Moon, Separating Water* and *Circular Chi Flow*. If you have a "spare tire," practice only *Lifting The Sky* and *Drawing The Moon* for about three months before adding the other two exercises.

# CHAPTER TWELVE

# For Those Who Have Aged But Would Like to Be Young

> Longevity is only desirable if it increases the duration of youth, and not that of old age. The lengthening of the senescent period would be a calamity.
>
> Alexis Carrel

### The Old Little Boy

Lao Ker Yew is nicknamed "Old Little Boy." At the age of thirty he looked sixty, but now he is sixty, and he looks thirty.

Old Little Boy was an opium addict for thirty years. He took the drug in a frantic attempt to numb his suffering, as conventional medicine could not help him. He literally suffered from about a dozen diseases, ranging from arthritis and rheumatism to ulcers and hernia.

Then, as a last resort, he practiced Chi Kung and his progress could be described as miraculous. One by one, his diseases disappeared. When he performed his *Induced Chi Flow* exercise, at an age when others could not bend down to touch their toes, his involuntary movements were so agile that only a gymnast could do them. Then for three months he passed black feces, which he knew were the toxic residues of opium he had accumulated for thirty years! After he had been thoroughly cleansed, he began to see visions of Gods and Buddhas. He dared not breathe a word about this for fear of being ridiculed. Indeed, initially he thought he had

gone crazy. Soon he discovered that he had psychic powers.

I know all this well because Lao Ker Yew is my student, and has been in close contact with me throughout these experiences. He still practices Chi Kung everyday, and has now developed to a high spiritual level. He often communicates non-verbally with higher beings, and sometimes in his "trance" he speaks Sanskrit, a language he does not even know!

### How Chi Kung Promotes Youthfulness

The main purpose of this chapter is to examine how Chi Kung can keep us youthful, even when we age. Many of my elderly students, both male and female, actually look and feel younger after they have practiced Chi Kung, reminding us that we are as young as we feel.

How does Chi Kung promote youthfulness? From the traditional Chi Kung perspective, the secret of youthfulness can be summed up in two words—health and vitality. Health includes physical, emotional, mental, and spiritual well-being; vitality means having the energy and zest for work and play. Hence, a person's chronological age may be sixty, but if he is fit and robust, eats well and sleeps soundly, is at peace with himself and with others, does his job vigorously, enjoys his leisure, and in most cases, still looks forward to sexual pleasures, then he is youthful.

The attainment of health and vitality through Chi Kung is traditionally explained through the concept of *jing, chi* and *shen*, which can be translated as "essence," "energy," and "spirit," and these are regarded as mankind's three treasures.

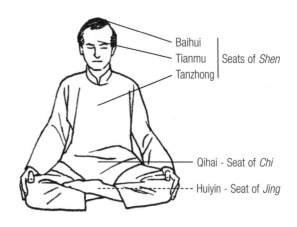

*Fig. 12.1 The Seats of Jing, Chi and Shen*

### The Concept of Jing, Chi and Shen

*Jing*, or essence, refers to the finest particles that constitute man. It is solid, but so fine that it is normally not visible to the eye. It forms the basis of all matter.

*Chi*, or energy, as we have seen, is our life force. *Chi* is formless, but Chi Kung masters have always emphasized that it has material reality. It is often manifested as physiological functions or the flow of electric impulses. Outside man's body, *chi* refers to cosmic energy.

*Shen*, or spirit, is man's consciousness, mind or soul, and it controls *jing* and *chi*. Your *shen* is the real You, covered by your *jing*, which in turn functions because of your *chi*.

Yet your *jing, chi* and *shen* form one whole unity. They are not different entities; they are intimately interrelated and are inter-convertible. For example, if a person's *jing* is inadequate, his *chi* and *shen* will be weak. It means that if a person is lacking in some substance (such as blood, flesh or hormones), his body may not function properly (physically or psychologically), resulting in a disturbed mind or consciousness.

The seat of a person's *jing* is at *huiyin*, the lower vital point between the genitals and the anus. The seat of a person's *chi* is at *qihai*, the middle vital point just below the navel. The seat of a person's *shen*, depending upon his spiritual development, is at his *tanzhong, tianmu*, or *baihui*, which are higher vital points located at the heart, the third eye and the crown of the head respectively.

These seats are focal points where *jing, chi*, and *shen* are accumulated. The whole body, being matter, is *jing*. The whole body is also *chi*, as it is fundamentally made up of energy. And the whole body, being permeated by consciousness, is *shen* too.

Practicing Chi Kung initially develops one's *jing*. Later *jing* is converted into *chi*. *Chi* may also be directly tapped from the cosmos by means of appropriate breathing exercises. Finally *chi* flows to the heart or head, and enhances our *shen*.

This means that at the initial stage of Chi Kung practice, we increase our appetite and add flesh and blood to our body. But we will not become fat, because our wonderful natural systems will allocate our mass to the right places. When the right amount of mass is attained, the excess mass will be broken down to provide energy for our bodily needs as well as for our work and play. Those who are large to begin with will have their excessive mass broken down when they start Chi Kung. We may also increase our energy by means of appropriate breathing methods, without first having to increase our mass. Continued practice of Chi Kung will enable energy to flow to our hearts or our heads, to develop our minds or our level of consciousness.

Hence, practicing Chi Kung gives us fit, healthy bodies, energy and vitality, as well as sound minds and enhanced consciousness to enjoy our youthfulness even when we age chronologically. This youthfulness is manifested in a strong yet supple spine, which provides an effective upright support for the physical body of *jing* or essence; a smooth, glowing complexion, which reflects a harmonious flow of *chi* or energy; and sparkling, lively eyes, which express the freshness of a calm yet alert mind.

## Overcoming the Causes of Aging

Like most Eastern people, the Chinese adopt a holistic approach to life, and in explaining why Chi Kung can promote youthfulness, they stress its effect on the whole person rather than on his parts. It is interesting to compare this holistic approach with the thematic approach generally used by the West, which attempts to understand the various processes in our body that contribute to aging.

The various theories suggested by Western scientists on aging processes are summarized by Pearson and Shaw in their enlightening book, *Life Extension: A Practical Scientific Approach*. They suggest that, "there are two basic classes of aging mechanisms, random damage and genetically programmed obsolescence." "Random damage" refers to all those damaging incidents, like the failure of the immune system to combat illness

and cross-linking of body tissues resulting in loss of flexibility, that lessen the quality and quantity of life. "Genetically programmed obsolescence" refers to the sudden but inevitable shutting off of a person's vital systems when he reaches his maximum possible life span. They propose that if we can eliminate random damage, we can live healthily to our genetically determined life span, probably around 120 years.

Pearson and Shaw describe the following theories put forward by contemporary scientists to explain aging: damage to DNA, failure of the immune system, cross-linked molecules, subversive free radicals, accumulated waste and decline of neurotransmitters. They also suggest that, within limits, we can even turn back genetically determined aging clocks to slow down our aging process.[8]

As I summarize these theories in the following sections, I also give my own theory of how Chi Kung overcomes the causes of aging. My theory may or may not be correct; but it is an attempt to explain, using Western terms, what actually happens, namely that practicing Chi Kung *does* slow down aging.

## Our Growth Blueprint and Immune System

DNA, or deoxyribonucleic acid, is the complex master molecule that contains the blueprint for a person's repair and growth. Damage to DNA is a major cause of aging. Scientists have discovered that the structure of a person's DNA changes when he or she is sick, but it reverts to its former structure when he or she recovers. Others have found that by passing an electromagnetic flow along an injured tissue or organ, they can speed up its regeneration or recovery.

Chi Kung masters have long helped patients to recover faster by channeling *chi* or energy to them; and the regenerative rate of Chi Kung practitioners is much faster than that of other people. I believe that a harmonious flow of energy in our bodies helps to realign our DNA structure to its proper pattern, thus preventing illness as well as eliminating random damage to the DNA, resulting in health and youthfulness.

Failure of the immune system causes diseases and aging, which reduce the quality and quantity of life immediately or in the future. For example, influenza, arthritis, multiple sclerosis or cancer occur because the immune system fails to check them. There is no doubt that Chi Kung strengthens our immune system, as explained in Chapter 6, thus minimizing or even eliminating another cause of random damage.

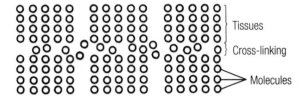

*Fig. 12.2 Cross-linking of Tissues*

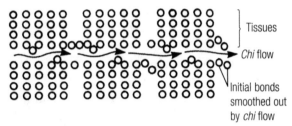

*Fig. 12.3 How Chi Flow Prevents Cross-linking*

### Cross-linking and Free Radicals

Cross-linking of body tissues is another major cause of aging. It occurs when large molecules in our bodies build undesirable chemical bridges across one another, causing damage like hardened arteries, wrinkled skin, and disturbed DNA structures. But when we let *chi* flow harmoniously in our bodies during Chi Kung practice, our stream of energy will smooth out the initial bonds, thus preventing the undesirable bridges from developing. This could explain why Chi Kung practitioners have smooth skin and supple arteries. Cross-linking and how it may be prevented by *chi* flow are shown diagrammatically in *figures 12.2* and *12.3*.

Free radicals are chemically reactive molecules or molecular fragments in our body. They are necessary in our normal metabolic reactions and in our defense system, where they react with and kill hostile foreign microorganisms. But if free radicals escape elsewhere, not only do they expedite aging processes by their subversive reaction (in the form of internal high-energy radiation), but they may also cause serious damage.

For example, if free radicals react with and damage the DNA, they bring about mutations, believed by many experts to be a major cause of cancer. If free radicals escape to the brain and react with oxygen there, they cause brain damage. So our body produces enzymes to control these free radicals, and this control is possible because of our effective feedback system. If there is some fault in the feedback system, free radicals may escape to speed up aging or cause more serious problems.

As explained in Chapter 4, Chi Kung enhances our feedback system, thus enabling us to produce the right amount of enzymes to keep the free radicals under control. Even if some free radicals escape, our *chi* flow can neutralize them, because the subatomic particles carried in the energy flow can react with the free radicals, thus eliminating their subversive radiation. Again this is just a theory at present, and I hope some researchers will test it. If those experts who regard the mutation of DNA as a major cause of cancer are right, then my theory explains why cancer patients can be cured after practicing Chi Kung.

## Waste Accumulation and Neuro-communication

Some scientists believe that aging is the result of the accumulation of toxic waste. Such waste is commonly called age pigments, like lipofuscin, ceroid and amyloid, which damage cells by blocking the flow of cytoplasm and interfering with diffusion, movement, and vital chemical reactions within the cell. Lipofuscin, for example, damages brain cells by clogging them so that vital nutrients cannot flow freely, causing senility. Chi Kung is an excellent means of removing toxic waste, thus promoting youthfulness.

Another important cause of aging is the decline of neuro-communication. Nerve cells communicate with each other by means of special chemicals called neuro-transmitters. The effective transmission of these messengers of the brain is essential for our delicate feedback system, which is responsible for the smooth functioning of all the activities necessary for living.

This neuro-communication is affected if impurities clog the nerves. Chi Kung overcomes this problem. When chi flows along the nerves, it clears them of impurities, known in Chi Kung terminology as cleansing the meridians. Hence, Chi Kung enhances our feedback system, which in turn helps to combat aging.

## Turning Back the Aging Clock

Within limits, Chi Kung can even turn back our aging clock! The turning on of each person's genetically determined clock is manifested by such symptoms as menopause, balding, and the loss of many regenerative capabilities. For example, a small child who loses the tip of a finger will sometimes grow a new one; adults have lost this capability.

The case histories of some of my Chi Kung students will surprise you. Some women men-struated again, although they had their menopause years before, and some men grew hair again although earlier they had been bald. The most surprising case, which has puzzled many doctors, concerned Choi, an insurance company manager.

A phalange (bone) of his finger was crushed in an accident. Choi was determined to have it back; so each time he practiced Chi Kung, he visualized its growth. After a few months he had a new phalange to replace his crushed one, and he proudly showed the finger with the new phalange to his Chi Kung classmates during a discussion!

There is a Chinese saying that, "One need not fear age if one's spine is still erect." A person is old if at thirty his spine is bent; whereas a person of sixty is still young if he comfortably holds his spine upright. The spine carries important networks of nerves to various parts of the body; an upright, relaxed spine facilitates the smooth flow of energy for total harmonious coordination. Practicing Chi Kung keeps our spines strong, supple and erect.

## Energy Flowing Up the Spine

The following exercise, known as *Long Breathing* in my Chi Kung school, stimulates the flow of energy along the full length of the spine from the *changqiang* vital point at the tip of the tailbone to *baihui* at the crown of the head. It is similar to *kundalini* in yoga.

This exercise should only be attempted if you have successfully completed *Abdominal Breathing* and *Submerged Breathing* (see Chapters 6 and 9).

1.  Stand upright and relax. Place your palms on your abdomen.
2.  Perform *Abdominal Breathing* about five times.

3. Then perform *Submerged Breathing* five times. As you breathe in, visualize cosmic energy flowing in through your nose and down to your *huiyin* vital point just near the anus. The in-flowing breath should be quite long, and your abdomen should rise gently.

4. Pause for a short while after breathing in. Then clench your toes and lift your anus (as if holding your anus to prevent feces coming out) as your *chi* travels the very short distance between the *huiyin* (before the anus) and the *changqiang* (after the anus).

5. Next, breathe out through your mouth and visualize *chi* flowing up your spine from *changqiang* to *baihui* at the crown of your head. Gently relax your toes and anus. Your abdomen will fall slightly as you breathe out.

6. Pause for a short while after breathing out. Repeat this procedure of breathing into the *huiyin-changqiang* area, and breathing out to the *baihui*, about twenty-six times. Remember to clench your toes and lift your anus, and do not forget two pauses.

7. Complete the exercise with *Standing Meditation*. Think of your *huiyin-changqiang* energy field, which is known as the "bottom of the sea" in classical texts. Visualize a beautiful full moon at the bottom of the sea, and let the pleasant moon energy gleam up at your body. Later, when this energy swells, enjoy almost

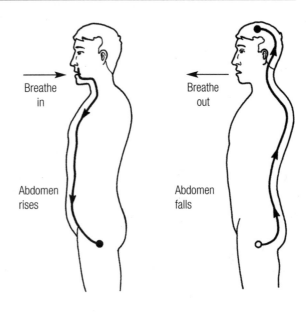

Breathe in

Abdomen rises

Breathe out

Abdomen falls

*Fig. 12.4 Chi Flow Direction in Long Breathing*

unconsciously the flow of energy up your spine. You will probably feel some pulsation at your *huiyin-changqiang* region, and later at your *baihui*.

Do not be surprised to experience a heightening of sexual excitement when your energy is focused at the *huiyin-changqiang* energy field. But do not abuse this feeling. Later, when your energy is focused at the higher energy field of *baihui*, you may find that you prefer mental or spiritual joys to carnal pleasures.

# PART FOUR

# The Internal Force of Martial Arts

# CHAPTER THIRTEEN

# *Chi Kung and Martial Arts*

If you want to soar to the heights and reach the depths of kungfu, you must practice Chi Kung; if you want to soar to the heights and reach the depths of Chi Kung, you must practice meditation.

Ho Fatt Nam

## *The Shaolin Successor and Uncle Righteousness*

The above is the best advice I have ever had in all my years of kungfu and Chi Kung training. It was given to me when my master, Sifu Ho Fatt Nam, taught me Chi Kung. "Sifu" is a respectful form of address for a master.

When the famous Shaolin Monastery in southern China was razed to the ground by the Qing army, one of its masters, the Venerable Jiang Nan, escaped, vowing that he would pass on the Shaolin arts to a selected disciple. After fifty years of wandering and searching, he finally passed them on to a young expert, Sifu Yang Fatt Khuen. Later, when he was in his seventies, Sifu Yang selected Sifu Ho as his successor.

Sifu Ho had practiced six different styles of kungfu as well as Malay Silat, and was a professional Siamese boxer before he learned Shaolin kungfu from Sifu Yang. Masters of several martial arts often challenged Sifu Ho, but he defeated them all.

Now he is better known as a Chinese physician, bonesetter, and acupuncturist, treating both royalty and commoners. But his greatest achievement, I believe, lies in meditation.

Another great kungfu master who greatly influenced me was Sifu Lai Chin Wah, who was more popularly and respectfully known by his nickname, "Uncle Righteousness." Uncle Righteousness was my first kungfu master, and he taught me like a son.

Sifu Lai's kungfu style was also southern Shaolin. He learned from three masters: Sifu Ng Yew Loong, Sifu Chui Khuen, and Sifu Lu Chan Wai. Sifu Ng's master was Sifu Chan Fook, a monk from the southern Shaolin Monastery.

Uncle Righteousness was an excellent kungfu fighter. In his day, when the fist, rather than the law, kept order in society, many people turned to him to settle disputes, like a magistrate. He told me people respected his decisions (which were always fair) because he had big fists to enforce them. He was also an accomplished bonesetter, but he did not become wealthy because he charged very little and sometimes gave money to the poor to buy food.

Among my masters, Sifu Lai Chin Wah and Sifu Ho Fatt Nam were the ones who contributed most to my kungfu and Chi Kung development.

It was my great privilege and honor, and a wonderful experience, to have been their disciple, learning from them not only the Shaolin arts but also the Shaolin philosophy of righteousness and compassion. I named my kungfu and Chi Kung school Shaolin Wahnam after them in appreciation of their kindness and generosity.

## A Little Knowledge is a Dangerous Thing

Chi Kung is closely connected with Chinese martial arts. Before 1950, when Chi Kung was taught exclusively to selected disciples, it was common for the general public in Asia to think of it as some form of advanced internal kungfu whereby the expert could injure his opponent without leaving any external mark, or take punches and even attacks with weapons without sustaining any injury. Since the 1980's, however, when the health aspect of Chi Kung began to be taught, many people have begun to think that it has nothing to do with martial arts!

Which of these two views is correct? They are, in fact, both right and both wrong. Some types of martial art Chi Kung, like *Iron Head* (in which you can break bricks with your head) and *Eagle Claw* (in which your grip can cause the opponent excruciating pain), are meant specifically for fighting and may be detrimental to health if the training is not done properly.

On the other hand, most medical Chi Kung types, like the *dao yin* exercises and *Induced Chi Flow* mentioned earlier, are specifically meant for curing illness and promoting health, and appear to have no connection with martial arts. Hence the view that martial arts Chi Kung and medical Chi Kung were mutually exclusive.

However, if we understand them more deeply, we see that they can be complementary, helping each other to achieve their special purposes. A proper training program of martial arts Chi Kung usually includes exercises that promote health. For example, before banging their heads against sandbags or jabbing their hands into granules—essential exercises for developing Iron Head and Eagle Claw—trainees must first practice Chi Kung exercises that make them healthy and fit, and protect their heads and hands with a covering of flowing *chi*, as well as clearing away any injury that they may sustain during training.

In the past, masters did not always explain this to their students when they taught them *Iron Head, Eagle Claw* and other specialized kungfu skills. This was part of a tradition to test their sincerity and perseverance. Those students who neglected these basic exercises would not be ready for the later hard conditioning; and others who unwittingly plunged into hard conditioning would injure themselves.

This explains why many laymen regard advanced kungfu as something mysterious. Not knowing about the need for the basic exercises, which often seem unrelated to the skills being sought, students may copy the masters' more obvious training methods, like hitting their heads against walls, and receive swollen heads instead of iron ones! They will never attain the masters' force or skill simply because they lack the basic foundation. This also means that in advanced kungfu, a little knowledge is often a dangerous thing. Without a master's supervision, students attempting advanced training are likely to injure themselves.

## Chi Kung for Health and Martial Arts

The standard of health and fitness demanded in kungfu training is generally higher than that required by most ordinary people. Most people would be quite contented if they were free from illness and pain, and be able to run a few steps to catch a bus. But this is not enough for a kungfu student; he should be able to endure vigorous exercises without feeling ill, take accidental punches from his sparring partners without feeling pain, and be able to spar for half an hour without feeling tired—abilities beyond most ordinary people. Hence, the health effects of martial arts Chi Kung are often greater than those of medical Chi Kung, because it is designed to attain a generally more demanding level.

On the other hand, Chi Kung of the medical school is very beneficial to martial artists, especially to those who heavily emphasize fighting techniques but are unaware of the concept of internal energy. More important than providing fitness (which martial artists have in abundance), good medical Chi Kung, like *dao yin* exercises and internal *chi* flow, ensures good health (which many martial artists may not have). Many martial artists have suffered insidious internal injury during sparring, and many are stressful, aggressive and irritable. Medical Chi Kung effectively cures internal injury and promotes emotional balance.

Furthermore, many medical Chi Kung exercises can enhance fighting skills. For example, *Lifting The Sky* (see Chapter 1) enables energy to flow to the arms and hands, making them more powerful internally. *Carrying The Moon* (see Chapter 2) strengthens the spine, promoting flexibility and agility. *Standing Meditation* (see Chapter 3) calms the mind, allowing martial artists to see their opponents' moves clearly. In advanced kungfu, *Induced Chi Flow* (see Chapter 4) is employed to enable the exponent to move fast and forcefully, yet without panting for breath.

Martial arts Chi Kung is sometimes known as "*hard* Chi Kung." However, the corresponding term, "*soft* Chi Kung," is seldom used to refer to medical Chi Kung, probably to avoid mistaken connotations.

If you have ever wondered why kungfu masters look gentle yet have tremendous force, or why women fighters in the past were graceful and fragile-looking yet had the power to match brutal male opponents, the answer lies in martial arts Chi Kung. Chi Kung also enables kungfu masters to maintain their power and stamina despite their age because it employs internal force, not just mechanical strength.

In kungfu, among other things, you can train to break a brick, to take punches without sustaining injury, to spar or fight for hours without panting for breath, and to jump high and run fast seemingly effortlessly. We shall now briefly examine the principles and training methods behind these skills. If you want to use these methods in your training, it is advisable to have supervision from a master.

### Pushing Mountains with Cosmos Palm

The method described here is part of an art called the *Cosmos Palm*, the art used by Sharifah to break a brick (see Chapter 2). Three factors are necessary: sufficient energy stored at the abdomen, the ability to channel this energy to the hand when it is needed, and a covering of energy around the palm to protect it.

First, practice *Abdominal Breathing* (Chapter 6) for at least three months to tap cosmic energy and store it at the abdomen. Then practice *Pushing Mountains* as follows.

1. Place your hands at your sides, at chest level with your palms facing forwards as in *figure 13.1*.
2. Gently push out your palms, as in *figure 13.2*, and simultaneously breathe out through your mouth. Do not use any strength, but visualize *chi* flowing from your back to your palms.
3. Next, gently bring back your palms, breathing into your abdomen and visualizing

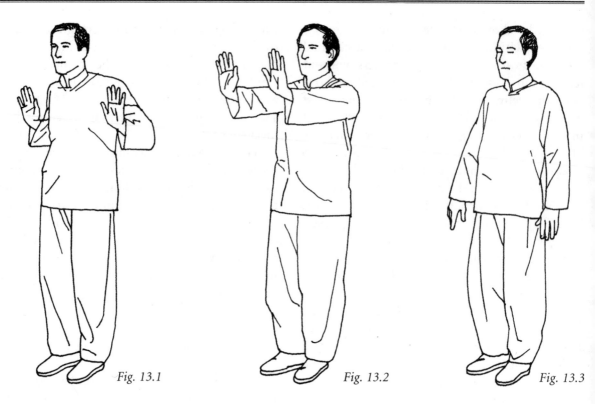

Fig. 13.1                                  Fig. 13.2                                  Fig. 13.3

*Figs. 13.1-13.2 Pushing Mountains*

cosmic energy flowing into you. Repeat this a few times.

4.  Then close your eyes, and as you push out, imagine that your *chi* is so powerful that you are pushing a mountain away. Practice this pushing about twenty to a hundred times, depending on your progress, for at least three months before performing the next stage.

5.  In the third stage, after *Pushing Mountains*, hold your palms stationary, as in *figure 13.2*, for about five to twenty minutes. Your palms should be at right angles to your forearms, your elbows straight, and your shoulders relaxed. Imagine that your palms are very powerful.

6.  Then drop your arms to your sides, with your palms facing backward, as in *figure 13.3*.

7.  Visualize two balls of energy at the center of your palms. You will feel your arms heavy, your palms very warm, your fingers tingling with power, and your whole body highly energized. In another three months, you will have developed *Cosmos Palms*. But remember: do not use *Cosmos Palm* imprudently—it can cause serious internal injury.

If at any time during practice you feel pain in your chest, you have been practicing wrongly, probably using your strength or breathing harshly. Correct your mistakes and the pain should go away. But if it becomes severe, you *must* stop practicing. If you persist, you may vomit or cough blood. If you do, your conventional doctor will say that there is nothing clinically wrong with you. *Induced Chi Flow* can solve this problem.

**Golden Bell, Lightness, and Tireless Fighting**

The two famous arts that enable the exponent to take punches and kicks and even attacks with weapons are *Iron Shirt* and *Golden Bell*. As it is highly probable that if you attempt them without a master's supervision, you will injure yourself, the following description is meant simply to satisfy your curiosity, *not* for you to attempt as self-training.

Chi Kung exercises are necessary to strengthen the body internally and to heal accidental injuries. In *Iron Shirt*, the exponent hits himself first with a bundle of sticks, then with bags of beans, and finally with bags of marbles or ball bearings. This spreads *chi* over his body as a protective cushion against external attacks. Not only does he not feel any pain, he actually enjoys the hitting—not that he has become masochistic, but the spreading of *chi* is quite a pleasant experience.

In *Golden Bell*, the exponent develops his energy internally and lets it radiate out to cover his body like a bell. Internal *chi* channeling and meditation are two important aspects in the training.

The skills of jumping high and of running far and fast are collectively known as the *Art of Lightness*; that is, the exponent has trained to become figuratively very light. One of my grandmasters demonstrated to my master, Sifu Ho Fatt Nam, his ability to jump a wall of about ten feet from a standing start. Unfortunately, this art is now lost to us, though we know the training techniques.

There are three levels of training in this *Art of Lightness*. In the first level, which is mechanical, the student goes about his daily activities with weights tied to his legs. He also digs a hole, and jumps in and out of the hole every morning and night. Each day he deepens the hole by scraping away a few bowls of soil.

In the second level, which uses *chi*, the exponent channels his *chi* to flow upwards as he jumps, making him feel very light. In the highest level, the mind level, the exponent, in a deeply meditative state, uses his mind to direct his physical body to rise. Though I have read about this feat by kungfu masters and spiritual leaders of the past, I have not yet been able to verify it from personal experience.

One useful method for developing the ability to run long distances with seemingly little effort is the *Art of a Thousand Steps* described in Chapter 8. Those who are proficient in this art should be able to spar or fight for hours without panting.

Another way to do so is to coordinate our breathing with our fighting movements. At the first stage of a kungfu set practice, for example, a student uses one breath for each kungfu pattern. Gradually he learns to use one breath for a series of patterns, performing them as if they were one long, smooth pattern. In this way, he can perform a long kungfu set made up of many patterns, with only a few breaths, and will still not be breathless at the end of the performance. Then he transfers this coordination skill to sparring or fighting.

This coordination will be enhanced if he employs *Small Universe Breathing*. Furthermore, if each time he breathes he can continually conserve thirty percent of this energy, and use only seventy percent for his fighting, he can fight for hours energetically. This breathing technique will be explained in the next chapter.

# CHAPTER FOURTEEN

# Shaolin: The Home of Kungfu and Meditation

All styles of kungfu owe their origins to Shaolin.
A popular kungfu saying

### The Shaolin Monastery and Bodhidharma

Shaolin kungfu is famous throughout the world. It is named after the Shaolin Monastery in China, which is sometimes known as "the foremost monastery on earth." There were actually two Shaolin monasteries, the original one in Henan Province in northern China, which still stands; and another in Fujian Province in the south, which was suspected of harboring revolutionaries and was razed to the ground by the army during the Qing Dynasty.

Founded in AD 495 by an Indian monk named Batuo, the northern Shaolin Monastery was an imperial temple where Chinese emperors throughout the ages ascended annually to pray to heaven on behalf of the empire. Many of the Shaolin monks were philosophers, poets, scholars, scientists, and retired generals seeking spirituality. There were some outstanding people among them, including the world-renowned Chinese astronomer Yi Xing, the famous pilgrim and translator Xuan Zang and the "wondrous" physician, Zhan Zhi.

In AD 527, the Venerable Bodhidharma, an Indian monk, arrived at Shaolin Monastery to teach meditation. In order to make the monks healthy and fit so that they were better prepared for their mental and spiritual training, Bodhidharma taught them two important sets of exercises: the *Eighteen Lohan Hands* and the *Classic of Sinew Metamorphosis*.

These exercises later formed the basis of Shaolin kungfu and Chi Kung. Bodhidharma is therefore honored as the first Patriarch of Shaolin kungfu. He is also the founder of Chan (or Zen) Buddhism.

The *dao yin* exercises described in this book, such as *Lifting the Sky*, *Carrying the Moon* and *Pushing Mountains*, are taken from *Eighteen Lohan Hands*, and many Chi Kung exercises for martial arts, like *Cosmos Palm*, are derived from *Sinew Metamorphosis*.

### The Classic of Sinew Metamorphosis

If you would like to "change" your muscles, sinews, and bones so that you are strengthened internally, then *Sinew Metamorphosis* is for you. There are twelve exercises, of which the following two are typical examples.

For the first one, stand upright and relaxed with your feet slightly apart, and your arms at your sides. Empty your mind of all thoughts.

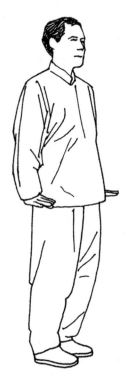

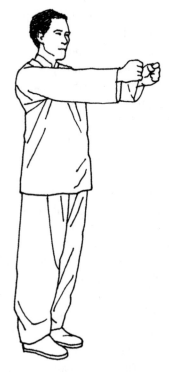

*Fig. 14.1 Sinew Metamorphosis (Flicking Fingers)*

*Fig. 14.2 Sinew Metamorphosis (Clenching Fists)*

Bend your wrists so that your hands are at right angles to your arms and your fingers point forward, as in *figure 14.1.*

While maintaining this posture, press down the heels of your hands, simultaneously raising your fingers as far as you can, forty-nine times. Do not worry about your breathing.

For the next exercise, which can be continued from the previous one or be performed separately, raise your arms to shoulders level in front of you. Keep them straight and clench your fists tightly, with the base of your fist pointing downward, as in *figure 14.2.* Clench and relax your fists forty-nine times. Again, do not worry about your breathing, but do keep an empty mind.

There is very little visible movement in these exercises, but you may feel your muscles, sinews and even bones moving internally. The exercises are extremely simple, but they produce marvelous results, strengthening not only your arms, but your whole body. Of course like all other exercises in this book, I do not expect you to take my word for this; practice them daily for a few months, and judge the effects for yourself.

### Hard and Soft: External and Internal

It is not an exaggeration to say that almost all types of techniques and force found in other martial arts are also found in Shaolin kungfu. But through lack of knowledge, some people have made the mistake of thinking that Shaolin kungfu is only hard, and never soft; that it is external, not internal. This misconception is caused by two factors. First, the earlier stages of Shaolin kungfu are comparatively hard and external; and because there is so much to learn, not many people have the patience or opportunity to progress to the more advanced levels, where much of Shaolin is soft and internal. Secondly, Shaolin demonstrations are often fast and powerful, suggesting that they are hard and external, at least compared with the gentle, graceful styles of *Taijiquan* (*Tai Chi Chuan*), *Baguazhang* (*Pa Kua Chang*) and *Xingyiquan* (*Hsing Yi Chuan*). Thus, it is common, though inaccurate, to classify Shaolin as the hard, external school of kungfu and *Taijiquan*, *Bagua* and *Xingyi* as the soft, internal schools.

"Hard" and "soft," "external" and "internal," are arbitrary, figurative terms. "Hard" refers to techniques or force that are generally dynamic, straight, and visibly powerful; "soft" to those that are generally graceful and circular, and whose power is hidden. Karate, for instance, is hard, whereas judo is soft. The word "soft" is actually a poor translation of the Chinese term *rou*, which never implies a lack of power, but it is the closest we can get. *Rou* force can in fact be more powerful than so-called "hard" force!

"External" refers to force that is developed through obvious, visual means, like lifting weights and striking poles; "internal" refers to force that is developed through abstruse, arcane methods, like channeling energy and visualization. A kungfu saying explains this poetically: internal force is acquired through the training of *jing* (essence), *shen* (mind), *chi* (energy); external force through the training of *jin* (sinews), *gu* (bones), *pi* (muscles). *Iron Palm*, for example, whose principal training method is jabbing the palm into granules and hitting it on sandbags, is external; whereas *Cosmos Palm*, whose principal method is *chi* channeling and visualization, is internal.

The classification into hard and soft force is relative and, as I have said, sometimes arbitrary. Prolonged training of a hard, external force can make it soft and internal, and vice versa.

It is helpful to know the difference between techniques (or *fa* in Chinese) and skills (*kung*).

Techniques refer to patterns and movements; they have form. Skills refer to how accurately, forcefully, and fast the techniques are executed; skills are formless. A very important kungfu principle warns that if you only learn techniques, but never develop skills, then your learning will be in vain, even if you carry on learning your whole life. The making of a master depends on the depth of his skills, not the extent of his techniques. In this chapter I describe some of the fundamental Chi Kung skills for developing internal force, as once practiced at the famous Shaolin Monastery.

### The Chi Kung Element in Kungfu

Although specialized Chi Kung force is usually introduced in the intermediate stage of Shaolin kungfu training, general Chi Kung is incorporated at the early stage, although often the student may not realize it. In southern Shaolin kungfu, for example, the very first thing a student does is to practice the *Horse-riding Stance*, (see *figure 14.3*), which is one of the most demanding tasks in kungfu training. My beloved master, Uncle Righteousness, made me practice just this one stance for several months before he taught me anything else. Among other things, practicing the *Horse-riding Stance* helps the student to store his energy at his abdomen.

In southern Shaolin kungfu, the student learns to let out different sounds explosively when he performs various kungfu patterns. These sounds help him to regulate his energy flow, as well as to strengthen different internal organs with their vibrations. For example, the sound "hert" is let out explosively from the abdomen (not from the throat as some novices mistakenly do) as one executes a punch. This sound not only adds internal force to the punch but also massages and strengthens the heart. The sound "yaaa" is used when executing a *Tiger Claw*, channeling internal

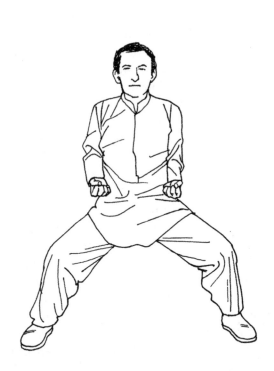

Fig. 14.3 The Horse-riding Stance

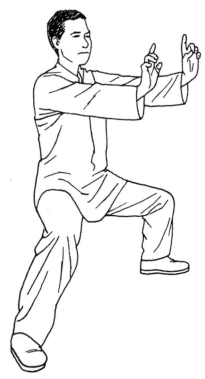

Fig. 14.3 The Golden Bridge

force to the fingers and vibrating the lungs.

The student is taught to coordinate his movements with correct breathing. For example, when he jumps or moves speedily, he breathes in rapidly with his chest, floating *chi* upward so that his movements become agile. As he strikes, he explodes out and sinks his *chi* to his abdomen, so that his movements are forceful and steady.

He also learns to execute a series of movements as if they were one long, smooth movement, and he does this in one breath. He learns when to hold his breath, when to breathe in or out quickly, and when slowly, letting out the breath like a long, thin thread. So the next time you hear a kungfu exponent making a lot of noise while fighting, remember that he is not trying to attract attention, or to scare his opponent; he is regulating his breathing to reinforce his fighting skills.

### Powerful Arms and Solid Stances

Southern Shaolin kungfu is well known for its development of powerful arms and solid stances. There is a kungfu saying that unless your opponent is an expert, if you have powerful arms and solid stances, you have won three-tenths of the battle. One of the best ways to achieve these is the hard Chi Kung known as *Golden Bridge*.

Take up the *Horse-riding Stance*, and hold both arms straight out in front of you at shoulder level, with your palms facing forward, your index fingers pointing up, your thumbs and all other fingers crooked at the second knuckle, in a typical Shaolin hand form called "One Finger Zen" (see *figure 14.4*).

Empty your mind of all thoughts and breathe naturally; this is a form of standing meditation.

The minimum requirement is to stand motionlessly in this position for five hundred counts or about ten minutes. If you want to count, do so at your abdomen. Do not think about how to do it; just count at your abdomen. Your back should be erect but relaxed, your thighs almost horizontal, and your hands at right angles to your wrists. If your posture is correct, do not be surprised if initially you cannot even last for a minute. Persevere daily, and hopefully in a few months' time, you will have achieved the minimum requirement of ten minutes, and you will be glad that you have put in the effort.

This technique may appear very simple, but it is one of the most tiring and most effective methods of developing internal force. When my kungfu students, many of whom are stronger and bigger than me, first spar with me, they find that my arms are like two pieces of hard wood. A few months later, after having practiced *Golden Bridge* consistently, they discover that my arms are no harder than theirs; but when they spar with beginners, their own arms seem to be like pieces of hard wood.

The internal force developed by *Golden Bridge* comes through the training of *jing*, or essence. Western physicists have worked out that if we strengthened every muscle in our arms, we would have enough power to lift a locomotive. In this hard Chi Kung exercise, we are strengthening some of these muscles at the molecular level. In the next exercise, we will train man's other two treasures, *shen* (mind) and *chi* (energy).

### The Forceful Small Universe

1  Stand upright and relax. Empty your mind of all thoughts.
2.  Place your palms on your abdomen.
3.  Clench your toes, lift your anus, and gently breathe through your nose into your chest (not your abdomen). Your abdomen will fall as you breathe in. Simultaneously, lift your tongue to touch your upper gum, where your upper teeth are set into your flesh. Visualize cosmic energy flowing into you, and your own vital energy flowing up your spine from the *huiyin* energy field (at the anus) to the *baihui* energy field (at the crown of your head).
4.  Hold your breath for a short while and focus your *chi* at *baihui*.
5.  Breathe out gently through your mouth and visualize *chi* flowing down your forehead, then down the front of your body into your abdomen. Your abdomen will rise as you breathe out. Simultaneously drop your tongue to touch your lower gum, and relax your toes and anus. But breathe out only about seventy percent of your breath.
6.  Gently hold the remaining thirty percent of your breath for a short while. Then gently "swallow" it into your abdomen, like swallowing some saliva. (In fact your mouth will probably be full of saliva, which is a good sign.)
7.  Visualize energy flowing down from your abdomen to your anus. Repeat the whole process about thirty-six times.
8.  Next proceed to *Standing Meditation* for about ten to twenty minutes. Gently visualize a ball of energy like a golden sun at the crown of your head, radiating wonderful energy to all parts of your body.
9.  End the exercise by warming your eyes and massaging your face.

This exercise completes the small universal *chi* flow in a relatively forceful way. Hence it is known as the *Forceful Small Universe*, and is very useful in martial arts Chi Kung. Later, when you are competent, you can perform this exercise with your feet about one and a half times your shoulders width apart, your knees slightly bent

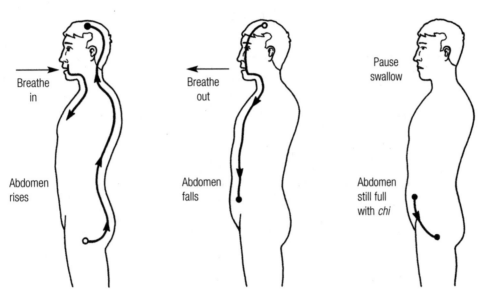

*Fig. 14.5 Chi Flow Direction in Forceful Small Universe*

and your arms hanging at your sides, as in *figure 14.6*. We call this the *Cosmos Stance* because we generally use it to tap energy from the cosmos. Some others call it the *Copper Bell Stance*, because it resembles a big copper bell.

*Forceful Small Universe* is an advanced Chi Kung method. You are advised not to practice it on your own, as serious injury can result if you do it wrong.

Chi Kung greatly enhances fighting skills. Unlike many other martial arts and various forms of physical exercises, martial arts Chi Kung allows a kungfu master to improve with age, because the force he develops is internal and increases with practice, rather than mechanical, which degrades with years. In my forties my Chi Kung practice helped me to beat opponents half my age and win the kungfu competition in the southern style division. My disciples, Cheng Shang Shou, also in his forties, and Goh Kok Hin, in his twenties, won in the remaining divisions of *Taijiquan* and northern style.

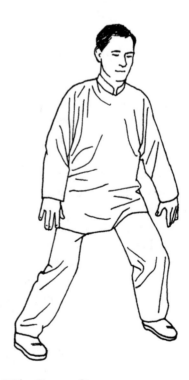

*Fig. 14.6 The Cosmos Stance*

# CHAPTER FIFTEEN

# Taiji: Energy and Poetry in Motion

T'ai-chi-Ch'uan connects the mind to the body, the consciousness to the subconscious and the individual to his environment. It ends the battles within you, eliminating tension and anxiety.

Bob Klein

## The Secret of Taijiquan

When you see someone practicing *Taijiquan* (the Romanized Chinese spelling for *Tai Chi Chuan*), you may mistake it for Chinese ballet. *Taijiquan* movements are graceful and rhythmic, suggesting poetry in motion. Yet *Taijiquan* is an exceedingly effective martial art.

How can such slow, gentle movements be used for fighting? Indeed, many people who practice *Taijiquan* today do not know the answer because they principally practice it for health. But to those great masters who first devised and developed *Taijiquan*, the health aspect was secondary or incidental; their primary aim was combat. Even now, if we examine *Taiji* forms and movements, we shall find that they are the way they are because of considerations of combat, not health. A *Taiji* performer moves in one particular way or holds one particular form, not because it promotes his health, but because it enables him to fight well.

This, of course, is not to deny the tremendous health benefits one will get from practicing *Taijiquan*. As explained in Chapter 13, almost all kungfu styles promote health and fitness because these are prerequisites for more demanding combat training. Because of its nature and philosophy, *Taijiquan* fulfils this health function better than most other styles. It is particularly useful for people who, for various reasons like age and illness, find the other more vigorous styles unsuitable.

But even looking at it from the health aspect alone, many *Taijiquan* students do not derive as much benefit as they should from their practice of the art. They gain something, of course, but the benefit would be much greater if they had a better understanding of the secret behind *Taijiquan*. And what is that secret? Chi Kung, of course.

## The Essential Role of Chi Kung

There are several reasons for calling *Taijiquan* one of the most beautiful martial arts in the world, and Chi Kung plays a crucial part in each.

While there are literally hundreds of kungfu sets in Shaolin, there is basically only one in *Taijiquan*. In the Yang style of *Taijiquan*, which is probably the most widely practiced today, the original set consisted of one hundred and eight patterns, which were repeated; its modern, simplified, version contains only twenty-four patterns. Yet these twenty-four patterns—if the exponent knows how to use them properly—are sufficient to meet any combat situation!

This streamlining of countless defense techniques into a few patterns which are still enough to handle any attack is a remarkable achievement. However, this is possible only if the exponent has internal force, for in many situations the *Taiji* techniques alone are not adequate. For example, if someone grips your wrist, you can make him release you by turning your wrist in such a way—as in Shaolin kungfu— that your hand presses hard on his wrist, causing him so much pain that he has to release his grip. This and similar techniques are not found in *Taijiquan*. So the *Taiji* exponent compensates for this lack with internal force. He may, for instance, use a typical *Taiji* circular arm movement, and at the appropriate moment exert an internal force which vibrates so powerfully that it dislodges the opponent's grip. This internal force is developed through Chi Kung.

Men and women of any age have an equal opportunity to excel in *Taijiquan*. In many martial arts, a young man has a clear advantage over an elderly woman, but not so in *Taijiquan*. This is because the force in *Taijiquan* is internal, and therefore is not affected by sex or age. Chi Kung is essential for building this force.

In many martial arts, the exponent pays the price of external force with bruised knuckles, roughened skin, and callused feet. The *Taiji* exponent can be powerful too; but not only does he not carry those telltale signs, but his Chi Kung training actually improves his complexion. Moreover, while many other martial artists, because of the nature of their training, tend to become more tense and aggressive, the *Taiji* exponent becomes more calm

and relaxed the more he trains. This is due to the harmonious effects of breathing and meditation exercises in *Taiji* Chi Kung.

*Taijiquan* not only provides you with a reliable form of self-defense, but heals you if you are sick and prevents you from becoming ill if you are already healthy. It is especially effective against organic disorders and emotional illnesses. You will enjoy these benefits even if you practice *Taijiquan* without any awareness of its Chi Kung aspects, but they will be greatly enhanced if you practice it with Chi Kung.

*Taiji* masters say that there are three levels of attainment in *Taijiquan*. At the first level the exponent can perform *Taiji* movements flowingly, and achieve health and fitness. At the second level he can apply the movements effectively to combat. At the highest level, as Bob Klein says in the quotation at the beginning of this chapter, he connects the mind to the body, the consciousness to the subconscious, and the individual to his environment. Chi Kung is helpful at the first level, necessary at the second, and essential at the third, where the exponent approaches the Taoist path to immortality.

### Why Are Taiji Movements Slow and Gentle?

Chi training in *Taiji* can be approached in two ways, and if you want the best, you should employ both. One way is intrinsic: *chi* training is incorporated into the *Taiji* set itself. The other is extrinsic: various Chi Kung exercises outside the *Taiji* set are used to develop internal force.

Have you ever wondered why *Taijiquan* is usually performed slowly and gently? It is because of intrinsic *chi* training. If the movements are fast and forced, energy will not flow smoothly. That is why *Taiji* instructors keep reminding their students not to use strength. The trouble is that they seldom explain how one can fight well without using strength, or why doing so will hamper the development of internal force.

In combat, just as in normal practice, the *Taiji* exponent does not use mechanical strength; he uses internal force. If he uses mechanical strength, he has to tense his muscles, which in turn will constrict his meridians and interrupt the internal energy flow. A *Taiji* exponent aims to be calm throughout—even when someone is endangering his life or those of his loved ones— so that *chi* flows endlessly inside him and provides him with stamina and internal force.

In his practice, he coordinates his movements with his internal *chi* flow. When he spreads his arms in the pattern *Separating Horse's Mane*, for example, his bodily movement must be such that his internal *chi* can reach his hands by the time they have reached the limit of their spread. If he moves his arms too fast, his *chi* flow may not follow quickly enough, with the result that his *chi* may only have reached the elbows (and be locked there) when the hand is already extended. And if he tenses his arm, or any part of his body, he blocks his flow of *chi*.

These slow, gentle movements are performed during practice. At an advanced stage, when his *chi* flow is as quick as he directs it with his mind, the *Taiji* exponent can be very fast. In fact, he has to be fast and forceful when he spars or fights.

### Intrinsic Chi Training in Taijiquan

Intrinsic *chi* training refers to developing internal force while performing a *Taiji* set or a series of *Taiji* movements. The pattern *Grasping Sparrow's Tail* is used as an example to illustrate the principles and method involved. It is assumed that the reader can perform the physical movements of the pattern competently; so explanation is only given for the breathing and visualization aspects. Please refer to the drawings in *figure 15.1*.

1. Stand upright and relax, with your mind clear of all irrelevant thoughts, *(a)*.
2. As you move your feet apart and raise your arms, *(b)*, breathe in gently through your nose. You may use chest breathing or *Abdominal Breathing* for this exercise.
3. As you lower your arms, breathe out gently through your mouth (or nose), *(c)*. Visualize *chi* flowing down your arms.
4. Breathe in at *(d)*.
5. As you move to *(e)*, visualize your *chi* flowing from your abdomen through your right shoulder and right elbow to your right hand, breathing out simultaneously.
6. Breathe in as you move through *(f)* to *(g)*, and visualize that you are charged with cosmic energy.
7. Breathe out as you move from *(h)* to *(i)*, and focus your energy at your right forearm.
8. As you lower your stance and move your body back slightly, *(j)*, breathe in, focusing your *chi* at both elbows (or at your wrists, if you are at an advanced level), and feel that you are firmly rooted on to the ground, although there should be more weight on your left foot.
9. Let your internal force explode (but do not use any strength) as you strike out, *(k)*, starting from your left heel, going through your waist, focused at your elbows (or wrists), and out of your palms into your opponent.

If you have accumulated cosmic energy at your abdomen to start with, your result will be faster and better. It is therefore recommended that you practice *Abdominal Breathing* (Chapter 6) for at least three months before you begin this intrinsic chi training in *Taijiquan*, if you have not already done so. A foundation of *Abdominal Breathing* to store cosmic energy is always an asset, irrespective of the style of martial arts you practice.

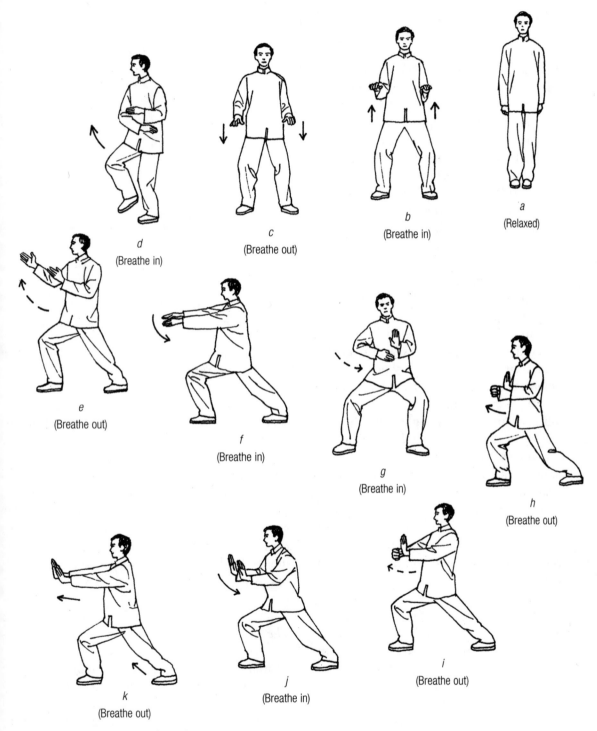

*Fig. 15.1 Grasping Sparrow's Tail*

## Vibrating with Internal Force

*Abdominal Breathing* is an extrinsic method. Another useful extrinsic method to develop internal force in *Taijiquan* is the *Three-Circle Stance*, sometimes called the *Taiji Stance* because it is so popular in *Taijiquan*. It is the *Taiji* counterpart of the *Golden Bridge* in Shaolin kungfu (see Chapter 14), and is used for training powerful arms and solid stances. It is softer than the *Golden Bridge*, and not as demanding, and the emphasis is more on the training of *chi* whereas the *Golden Bridge* emphasizes *jing* (essence) more.

1.  Stand with your feet about one and a half times your shoulder width apart and bend your knees slightly.
2.  Hold your arms at chest level in front of you, with your elbows and wrists slightly bent to form a circle. Your fingers should be held loosely apart, with thumbs and index fingers forming a small second circle.
3.  Pull in your abdomen slightly and hook in your knees as if you were holding a ball with your thighs, thus forming the third "circle" (although it may not look much like one).
4.  Clear your mind of all thoughts. Your eyes can be open or closed.
5.  Stand motionless in this *Three-Circle Stance* for as long as you can. The minimum requirement is one thousand counts or about twenty minutes.

Do not worry if, after practicing for some time, parts or the whole of your body vibrate or shake vigorously. This is a manifestation of the kungfu principle that extreme stillness generates motion. It is caused by the vigorous internal flow of energy, and is a sign that you have developed internal force. Many people find it hard to believe that such a simple technique can develop force, or

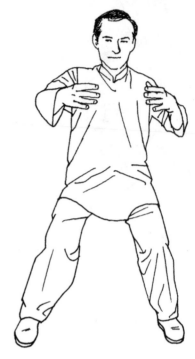

*Fig. 15.2 The Three-circle Stance*

that the body can vibrate involuntarily, until they try it out themselves.

When you have acquired internal force, you can use it in many different ways. You can use it to improve your *Taijiquan* performance or sparring. You can also channel it out of your body, as in *chi* channeling therapy, where the therapist transmits *chi* to a patient to help him relieve pain or cure illness. And of course you will use it unconsciously in your daily work and play.

## The Gentle Small Universe

Your *Taijiquan* can be improved tremendously if you can attain the *Small Universal Chi Flow*, or the *Small Universe*. In the past, attaining the *Small Universe* was regarded as a great achievement that called for a grand celebration.

There is a traditional Chi Kung saying that if you achieve the breakthrough of the *Small Universe*, you will eliminate hundreds of diseases; if you achieve the breakthrough of the *Big Universe*, you will live for a hundred years. The attainment of the *Small Universe* is highly valued by martial artists, because it speeds up the development of internal force, and acts as a safety valve to prevent internal injury caused by training wrongly.

There are two approaches to the *Small Universe:* the forceful and the gentle. The *Forceful Small Universe* is explained in the previous chapter; here we will look at the *Gentle Small Universe*.

You must be proficient at *Abdominal Breathing* (Chapter 6), *Submerged Breathing* (Chapter 9) and *Long Breathing* (Chapter 12) before attempting the *Gentle Small Universe*.

1. Stand in the *Cosmos Stance* (Chapter 14), with your palms gently on your abdomen.
2. Start by practicing *Abdominal Breathing, Submerged Breathing* and *Long Breathing* about ten times each.

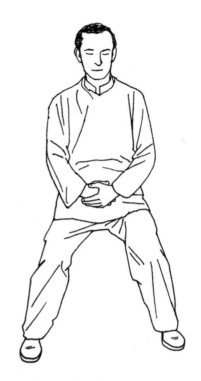

*Fig. 15.3 Gentle Small Universe in the Cosmos Stance*

3. With the tip of your tongue touching your upper gum, gently breathe through your nose into your abdomen, visualizing that you are tapping wonderful cosmic energy from the universe and storing it at the energy field there. Your abdomen will rise as you breathe in.
4. Pause for a short while to feel the cosmic energy at your abdomen.
5. Breathe out gently through your mouth, with your tongue now touching your lower gum, where your lower teeth are set in your flesh, and visualizing your vital energy flowing from your *qihai* vital point (at the abdomen), to your *huiyin* (before the anus), across to *changqiang* (at the coccyx), up the spine to baihiui (at the crown of the head), down the front of your face and out of your mouth (see *figure 15.4*). Your abdomen will fall as you breathe out.

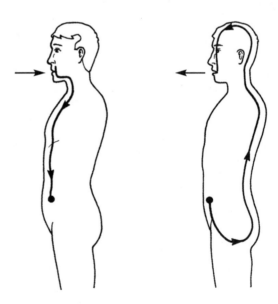

*Fig. 15.4 Chi Flow Direction in Small Universe*

6.  Pause for a short while after breathing out.

7.  Repeat this breathing into the abdomen, and breathing out round the body and out of the mouth—thus completing the *Small Universe*—about twenty times. Gradually increase the number of times as you progress. Later, you can start the exercise with this gentle small universal breathing, without the need to perform the preliminary *Abdominal Breathing*, *Submerged Breathing* and *Long Breathing*.

8.  Next, bring your feet together for *Standing Meditation*. Close your normal eyes, and open your *Third Eye*, which is situated just above the spot between your normal eyes. Just gently think of your *Third Eye* open. Then look inwardly, or figuratively, into your abdomen, and see (or imagine) a pearl of energy at the energy field there. Take a few minutes to enjoy the glow of this beautiful pearl subconsciously.

9.  Visualize a stream of energy issuing from the pearl, and flowing along the path of the *Small Universe*. Subconsciously enjoy this small universal *chi* flow for a few minutes.

10. Then visualize the pearl of energy again. Feel its glow and warmth, and let its energy radiate to every cell in your body, bringing vitality and life.

11. Complete the exercise by warming your normal eyes before opening them, and massaging your face.

All the visualization must be done gently—very gently. Do *not* insist on any vision if you cannot see it. If visualization is difficult, just thinking of it may suffice. Like the *Forceful Small Universe* in the previous chapter, it is not advisable to attempt this exercise without supervision from a master.

# PART FIVE

# The Training of the Wondeful Mind

# CHAPTER SIXTEEN

# Improving Academic Performance through Chi Kung

A few years ago, meditation usually meant to most a "religious" reflection....But in the East, meditation had long been practiced as a mode of achieving consciousness on various levels of awareness, and the coming to the West of this teaching has brought about a new realization of the potential of this form of approach to that which is inner, higher or spiritual.

Michael J. Eastcott, 1969

### Why Chi Kung Improves Academic Performance

Here is some good news for parents: Recent research carried out in schools, colleges, and universities in China shows that practicing Chi Kung helps students to improve both their sporting and their academic performance. How Chi Kung benefits sportsmen has been explained in Chapter 8 in Part Three. Part Four explains how Chi Kung develops internal force, which is useful to both sportsmen and scholars. In this section of the book we examine how Chi Kung trains the mind.

It is not only the young who will benefit; Chi Kung improves the mental faculties of adults too. For example, research conducted at the Bai Diu En Medical University on thirty-seven pensioners between fifty-five and seventy-seven years old showed that by practicing Chi Kung for twenty days, their concentration improved remarkably. And research at China's Science College Biophysics Research Center shows that practicing Chi Kung prevents the degeneration of fluid intelligence in elderly people, thus delaying or preventing senility.[9]

There are many reasons why Chi Kung improves academic performance. First, it enhances physical, emotional and mental health, enabling the student to give of his best.

Secondly, it provides abundant energy, which is frequently needed even more in mental than physical work. Many students get their energy from the food they eat. But high-energy food can be quite expensive, and even if the students can afford it, it cannot be taken continuously, for an excess even of good food becomes poison in their body.

Even if the right amount of food is taken, it takes some time to digest and absorb, which explains why eating a rich, heavy meal just before sitting for an examination is a burden rather than an aid. But cosmic energy, which is probably the purest and finest energy, is free and immediate. A candidate who has just taken energy from the cosmos will find himself energetic and alert in an examination.

For ordinary students, the energy needed for mental work is derived from oxidation of food, which also produces waste products. If these waste products are not cleared efficiently, they may clog the brain cells, blocking the flow of nutrients to the cells as well as the smooth flow of mental impulses. Clearing these waste products is usually done by deep breathing brought about by recreational exercise.

But if we take the energy needed for mental work directly from the cosmos instead of from food, there may be little or no waste as there is no need for any oxidation of food. Moreover, Chi Kung is more effective than recreational exercise in clearing waste products, because it directly employs the best breathing methods for this purpose. Moreover, it also brings vital energy to the brain cells. It therefore improves the freshness of the mind.

### Focused Mind and Visualization Ability

The mind of a student who practices Chi Kung is also better focused than that of an ordinary student. Many people cannot concentrate because their untrained minds, to use a Chinese saying, are like monkeys and wild horses, running everywhere. Chi Kung training brings these "monkeys and horses" under control, and develops a focused mind.

Furthermore, a Chi Kung student can use his mind more efficiently than an untrained student. His ability to visualize, which is developed through Chi Kung practice, not only enables him to see problems clearly in his mind, but also to consider possible solutions for his problems through visualization.

Chi Kung provides students with a rare opportunity to enter different levels of consciousness, and to explore different levels of reality. In deep meditation, they may have access to the Universal Mind (to be discussed in later chapters), from which they can draw great moments of inspiration and creativity.

With such an impressive array of factors in its favor, it is no wonder that Chi Kung greatly improves academic performance. The Chinese are so excited by this discovery that since 1986, when Professor Qian Xue Sen, the father of the Chinese rocket, actively promoted Chi Kung as a means to expand the intellect, they have introduced a new genre into the classification of Chi Kung, intellectual Chi Kung, although the function of Chi Kung in the training of the mind was long recognized in the past.

### Mental Development in Chi Kung

In all the major schools of Chi Kung, mental development is an important function, especially at the advanced levels. But this mental aspect is present at all levels, even though many beginners may not be aware of it. In the medical school of Chi Kung, the unity of mind and body is always emphasized. The *Nei Jing*, regarded by many as the final authority on Chinese medicine, advises: "Discard all irrelevant thoughts, breathe in cosmic energy, so as to open your mental faculties."

In martial arts Chi Kung, keeping the mind empty or focused on only one thought is an essential factor. The highest achievements in Shaolin or *Taiji* kungfu occur through meditation, which is a process of mind training. Confucian Chi Kung stresses that silence gives birth to intellect. The following advice from the great Song scholar, Chu Hsi (Zhu Xi in romanized Chinese), has become a Confucian maxim: "Spend half the day on meditation, and the other half on study."

In Taoist and Buddhist Chi Kung, the highest level is meditation, the golden path to spiritual fulfillment (see Chapter 21). It must be emphasized here that terms like "Confucian," "Taoist," and "Buddhist" are philosophical or historical rather than religious, and their methods can thus be used by people of any religion. At a lower level, where the mind, rather than the spirit, is emphasized, the Taoists advocate "the flow of essence to nourish the mind," which describes a fundamental principle in using cosmic energy to open mental faculties, as in *Small Universe* Chi Kung. The Buddhists teach that "stillness creates wisdom," which is a concise way of saying that through meditation one can attain fantastic mental abilities, including psychic powers.

Of the various schools of Chi Kung, the Confucian is the most immediate in promoting academic achievements. But you are in for a surprise if you think that their methods and philosophy merely help students to pass examinations with flying colors—although they do that as well as can be seen by the number of Confucian scholars who gained distinctions in China's imperial examinations for the Civil Service. However there is more to it than that—many of their ideas preceded modern science.

## Confucian Chi Kung and Intellectual Development

Some people have a mistaken picture of Confucius (Kong Fu Zi in romanized Chinese) as an old man so loaded with book learning that he could hardly run. Actually, he was well versed in the "six arts"—rites, music, archery, horsemanship, literature and mathematics—besides being a Chi Kung expert. He said that *chi* affects not only our physical health but also our emotions, and that if our *chi* is full, it changes into *shen* (mind), enhancing our intellectual work.

Mencius (Meng Zi), regarded by Confucians as second only to Confucius in greatness, said that the physical body is actually a body of energy—and he said it more than two thousand years before our modern scientists. Mencius' most quoted statement is: "I am good at nurturing energy taken from the wide cosmos." He said that

the aim of filling ourselves with cosmic energy is to enable us to be righteous; one who has mean or evil intentions will not benefit from the righteous energy of the universe. Here Mencius was propounding the philosophical ideal of Confucian Chi Kung, the attainment of high moral values, which is different from the spiritual orientation of the Taoist and Buddhist schools.

Another great Confucian master, Hsun Tzu (Xun Zi), said that the secret art of regulating energy and developing mind was none other than maintaining high moral values, learning from a good master, and being steadfast in our practice. Many of the great Tang poets like Po Chu Yi (Bai Ju Yi), Tu Fu (Du Fu), Liu Zong Yuan and Wang Wei practiced Chi Kung, which was often reflected in their work. A poem of Liu Zong Yuan says:

> I heard of a secret art from a sage
> Accumulating energy in the middle of night.
> His breathing gentle, deep and slow,
> Down to his roots flows his energy with might.

This short verse reveals a favorite time and a popular technique of the Tang scholars in their Chi Kung practice. A favorite time is between 11 PM and 1 AM, which Chi Kung masters regard as a time of blossoming energy. A popular technique is gentle, deep, slow breathing right down to the heels, known as *Heel Breathing*.

Su Tung Po (Su Dong Bo) and Chu Hsi were two of China's greatest scholars who owed their success mainly to Chi Kung, and who actively promoted the art. Su Tung Po believed that the fundamental art of longevity was "fetus breathing," which refers to internal breathing without the use of nose or mouth. Chu Hsi said that, in mediation, we first eliminate all thoughts, and then we look at our thoughts at a heightened level of consciousness. We shall learn a similar technique for solving problems and enrich creativity in the next chapter.

### *Discoveries of Confucian Scientists*

The discoveries of the two great Confucian scientists of the Song Dynasty, Zhang Dai and Shao Yong, whose work was mentioned in Chapter 3, were awe-inspiring. Zhang Dai was convinced that energy fills every part of the infinite cosmos, and acts as a universal medium connecting everything. Hence he said, "A sage knows by intuitive wisdom, not limited by what he sees and hears only. In the whole universe, there is nothing that is not me." The discovery of the universal energy field by scientists today confirms the truth of his statement. He also emphasized the maxim of Confucian Chi Kung philosophy. He stressed that:

> If our heart is at peace, our whole body of energy is at peace. If our heart is righteous, our whole body of energy is righteous.

While Zhang Dai talked about the infinite cosmos, Shao Yong described the infinitesimal subatomic world. Both also expounded the great importance of the human heart or consciousness. In a poem called "Observing Change," Shao Yong said:

> Another body, a particle of matter has,
> This body, a cosmos of great delight.
> To know the nature of everything,
> Its three aspects be separated with might.
> Form and function, this heaven's made;
> The world man sees only from his mind.
> The great change, heaven and man abide,
> But man misses the void of great sublime.

It is only now, when modern physics has revealed to us the mystery of the subatomic world, that we can fully appreciate the depth of Shao Yong's perception. With hindsight, we now know that the "three aspects" refer to what modern scientists call neutron, proton and electron; "heaven" refers to the micro-cosmos of the particle; "form and function" refers to the particle-wave phenomena; and "void" refers to the undiffer-entiated spread of the energy field which, because of the limitation of our naked eyes, we see as differentiated, individualized entities.

The obvious question is: how did these ancient masters know about the infinite cosmos and the infinitesimal particle? The answer is through Chi Kung meditation.

In another poem called "Where is the Abode of Gods?" Shao Yong, described his mystical experience of deep meditation:

> Where is the abode of gods?
> In my chamber, now and here.
> Around me spreads the infinite.
> My heart feels cool and clear.
> In stillness I experience the void
> Containing the sun and moon.
> When this reality is perceived,
> Mere philosophy can be discarded soon.

Gao Pan Long, a Confucian scientist of the Ming Dynasty, gives us some idea of Confucian meditation in his "Song of Silent Sitting:"

> Silent Sitting is not from Tao or Chan.
> We developed our art from sages wise.
> Subduing emotions, righteous heart is born.
> Cosmic energy swells ere thoughts arise.
> Ours can be explained by ordinary means.
> There's no mystery nor supernatural way.
> When one day the supreme truth you see
> Enlightenment is natural you'll surely say.
> The infinite becomes clear and still.
> No other way to accomplish this skill.
> The cosmos has pulsated since ancient time.
> The sun and moon up the sky still climb.
> No need for elixir made by saints
> Nor talks of the void by the wise.
> Where our Confucian secret lies
> Is before thoughts and feelings arise.

Although he suggests that Confucian meditation is different from that of the Taoists and Buddhists, his technique is similar to that used in Chan (or Zen) meditation—by eliminating all thoughts and emotions, we see reality in moments of enlightenment.

## *The Art of Opening Intellect*

If you want to leave enlightenment till later and prefer to enhance your intelligence now, the following exercise is invaluable. It has been promoted by Yan Xin, who although only about forty, is one of the greatest Chi Kung masters in the world today. Most of you will find it hard to believe what he has done. In his public Chi Kung seminars, attended by thousands of people, he transmitted *chi* to the audience while he was talking, causing many people to experience involuntary *chi* flow that often cured their illnesses instantly! In a series of controlled experiments in 1986 and 1987, he transmitted *chi* over great distances (ranging between 7 km and 2000 km) to change the molecular structures of various liquids. These experiments were done not in private houses, watched by amateurs, but in the prestigious Qing Hua University of Beijing, supervised by some of China's most respected scientists.

1. Sit comfortably with your legs firmly on the floor and your back upright.
2. Place your left palm about two inches in front of your *zhongji* vital point (about midway between your navel, and your genitals).
3. Place your right palm about two inches in front of your left nipple. Make sure that your shoulders and elbows are relaxed.
4. Breathe naturally. Silently count your inhalations 120 times. Simultaneously visualize a warm, glowing light flowing from your *huiyin* vital point (at your anus) to your *baihui* vital point (at the crown of your head).

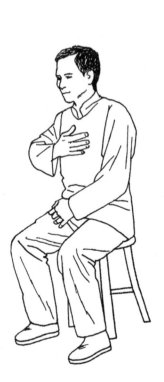

*Fig. 16.1 Enhancing Intelligence*

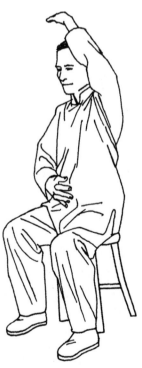

*Fig. 16.2 Anti-clockwise Rotation Above Baihui*

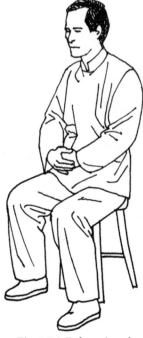

*Fig. 16.2 Enhancing the Middle Energy Field*

5.  Silently count your exhalations, also 120 times. Visualize *chi* flowing out of your *yuzhen* vital point (the midpoint between your ears at the back of your head). The breathing should be slow, gentle and long. Also visualize light from your palm shining on your heart.

6.  After counting the inhalations and exhalations 120 times each, gently place your left hand over your *baihui*, and slowly rotate it in an anticlockwise direction forty-nine times. Visualize *chi* being drawn back from the *baihui*.

7.  Gently bring your left hand from your head down your body to your abdomen, bringing *chi* from *baihui* to *qihai* (about two or three inches below the navel).

8.  Place your left hand about two inches above *qihai*, and your right hand on your left, and visualize *chi* focusing at this energy field at the abdomen.

9.  Complete the exercise with facial massage followed by brisk walking.

If you are a parent and you want your children to excel academically, then Chi Kung can provide the means. If you are a student yourself, with your intellect open, you can not only expect your performance to improve, but you can reasonably aim for academic excellence. The next chapter provides further information to help you achieve this goal.

# CHAPTER SEVENTEEN

## The Chi Kung Way to Inspiration and Creativity

There was a time when meadow, grove, and stream,
The earth, and every common sight,
To me did seem
Appareled in celestial light,
The glory and the freshness of a dream.
　　　　　　William Wordsworth, *"Intimations of Immortality"*

### Our Wonderful Mind

What did Solon, Lao Tzu, Patanjali, Nostradamus, Leonardo da Vinci, Wordsworth, Beethoven, and Edison all have in common? They all accomplished their greatest works while they were in meditation. They might not have sat in a formal meditation posture, but they were in a meditative state of mind, different from their normal selves, when they attained their great achievements. Indeed, it has been said that all great works of art, science, philosophy and religion were accomplished when the creators were cut off from ordinary affairs, in a state of sublime consciousness, when they were in contact with the Universal Mind.

Although most people differentiate the mind from the brain, controversy still persists as to whether the mind exists separately from the brain. Most people agree that the mind is non-material, non-physical and infinite, whereas the brain is visible, organic and limited to a definite structure. However, some experts argue that the mind is a convenient term to use when referring to the function of the brain. Richard Restak, a well-known neuroscientist, says:

> There is simply nothing to prove that anything exists other than the brain interacting with some aspects of external or internal reality. For this reason it should not be surprising that brain scientists haven't yet discovered the "seat of the mind." It is not likely that they will ....
>
> Mind, consciousness, and "self-awareness" represent an interesting degree of complexity in the structure and operation of the brain. [10]

It was probably opinions such as this which prompted Bertrand Russell to remark that when a neurosurgeon operated on somebody's brain, all he saw was his own brain. Nevertheless, other notable neuroscientists like Wilder Penfield and Sir John Eccles believe that the mind and the brain are distinct entities.

The separate disciplines of psychiatry and neurology are a good indication of the general belief in the distinction between mind and brain. Psychiatrists attend to mental illness, whereas neurologists treat brain disorder. Our daily use of language is also indicative of this distinction. We say, "I have changed my mind," knowing full well that we still have the same brain. We assure our friends that our thoughts are with them, although our brain is still in our own body.

Throughout the ages, meditation has involved the training of the mind, but it has never been bothered with a detailed study of the brain. Even without any deep understanding of the structure or functioning of the brain, meditators can still accomplish great things.

No one has actually seen an atom, but no informed person would seriously doubt its existence because without it many real events or processes would be meaningless, if not impossible. Similarly, no one has physically seen the mind, but there have been many proven cases and documented facts of supernormal abilities whose explanation would be meaningless without the concept of mind as a distinct entity from brain.

### Various Concepts of Mind in Chi Kung

The concept of mind in Chi Kung is much influenced by medical, Taoist, and Buddhist philosophies. In Chinese, "mind" may be expressed as "heart," "spirit," "soul," and "consciousness." In Chinese medical philosophy, the seat of the mind is in the heart, not in the brain. That is perhaps why Richard Restak is unable to find it when he operates on the brain! It is interesting to note that many great peoples in history have referred to the heart, and not the brain, as the seat of the mind; for example, the Indians, the Egyptians, the Persians, the Arabs, the ancient Greeks and Romans, as well as the medieval Europeans.

It is a mistake to think that these great peoples had no knowledge of the organ which modern doctors call the brain. The term "brain" is found in old Chinese texts. The *Nei Jing*, for example, contains some accurate information about the brain. Much later, but still earlier than conven-

tional Western medicine, the great Chinese physician of the Qing Dynasty, Wang Qing Ren, gave detailed descriptions of its anatomy and physiology.

Disease of the mind, known as disease of the heart in Chinese, concerns both mental and emotional disorders. The Chinese do not make a distinction between neurological and psychological diseases. To the Chinese physician, all diseases are interrelated. Hence, if a person is physically ill or emotionally disturbed, his mind will be weak. Physical and emotional health is a prerequisite for training the mind for intellectual activities.

In Taoist Chi Kung, mind is usually interpreted as "soul" or "spirit." The progress of Taoist Chi Kung from the elementary to the advanced levels can be summarized as the training of essence (*jing*), of energy (*qi*), and of mind or spirit (*shen*) (see Chapter 12). These three "treasures" of man are integrated, although the real self is the mind. Essence and energy serve to nourish the mind.

A Taoist Chi Kung principle states that if essence is full, energy is plentiful; and if energy is plentiful, mind is rich. Hence, to achieve a developed mind, it is necessary to have full essence (such as a fit and healthy body), and plentiful energy (such as vitality for work and play).

Insight, inspiration, creativity and intellectual activities come easily to a developed mind. Though these abilities are useful and make worldly life rewarding, they are not the primary aim of a Taoist. His ultimate aim is to free himself from his physical body, even while in this life, thus realizing "immortality."

Like the Taoist, the Buddhist strongly emphasizes developing his mind, and when his mind is developed to a very high level, he is capable of not only enhanced creativity and inspiration, but also supernormal powers, which laypeople call miracles. Like the Taoist, again, acquiring these powers is never his main aim;

they merely come as by-products, which are even regarded as a hindrance by many masters.

The Buddhist concept of mind is perhaps best expressed as consciousness, and in Chinese it is referred to as heart. The Buddhists, like many other peoples of ancient cultures, believe that every being, animate or inanimate (in the Western sense), has mind—centuries before modern scientists like Henry Stapp and E. H. Walker suggested that photons have consciousness.

The force of mind is supreme, and it is the primary force of the universe. The mind is centered in the heart, and it permeates every cell of the body. The brain has no particular significance in its attachment to the mind. It is the mind that really perceives: the sense organs merely act as connecting agents. Whatever we do is really what the mind does; the body cannot do anything on its own.

The aim of Buddhism is to purify the mind, to cleanse it of all the defilements it has gathered during its journey through countless lives. When the mind is pure, it sees reality as it really is. This is enlightenment, and it is attained through meditation.

Obviously, at the elementary and even the intermediate stages, the Taoist and the Buddhist concepts of mind are not significant. Indeed, when I first talked about mind in this context, many people accused me of mystifying Chi Kung because they understood it only at its more elementary, physical level. But if they had investigated the classical texts describing advanced Chi Kung—which were kept secret in the past—they would have found that Chi Kung techniques at the highest levels all deal with mind.

We can still achieve health and fitness by practicing Chi Kung without being aware of the mental aspects. But if we want to know why Chi Kung can enhance insight and creativity, or enable us to perform miraculous feats and how, we need to understand these esoteric concepts of mind.

## The Marvels of the Subconscious Mind

Taoist Chi Kung refers to two classifications of mind—primordial and intellectual—whereas Buddhist Chi Kung talks about entering four major levels of consciousness in meditation. These concepts correspond to the conscious and subconscious (or superconscious) mind in Western terminology. The conscious and the subconscious are not two minds, but two aspects of the same mind.

The conscious mind is the waking, working mind. Its most important function is reasoning: it enables us to think, to choose, and to make decisions.

The subconscious mind does not think. It has no reasoning power, but it performs other very important functions. It regulates your breathing, adjusts your blood pressure, organizes your digestion, and performs all the psychological functions necessary for living. It is also the seat of your emotions and the storehouse of your memory. All that you have learned and experienced in your whole life (even in past lives, as shown and confirmed by hypnotic regression) are recorded in the subconscious mind.

It is the working of the subconscious mind that enables artists, scientists, philosophers and all great men to produce their greatest works. The subconscious mind transcends time and space; its working gives us extrasensory perceptions like telepathy, clairvoyance, and precognition, and enables us unconsciously to draw on information that has been learned and organized in a different temporal or spatial dimension. William James, the father of American psychology, said that the power that moves the world is in the subconscious mind. Our subconscious minds have infinite knowledge and wisdom, as they are our link with the omniscient, omnipresent Universal Mind.

### The Universal Mind

The Universal Mind is known by many other names, such as Universal Consciousness, Ultimate Reality, Supreme Being, Tao, Grand Ultimate, Brahman, and God. With the breathtaking revelations of new physics—and without the slightest disrespect to the religious— we might refer to the Universal Mind as the grand undifferentiated energy field.

The Universal Mind is beyond space and time. It permeates everything, from the subatomic particle to the infinite universe. The subconscious mind is a part and an expression of the Universal Mind. The Universal Mind is one continuous reality: the duality, individuality and differen- tiation we see in the myriad things and beings around us is an illusion caused by the limitations of our senses. In other words, at our ordinary level of consciousness, we perceive objects as different and separate from one another. This to us is real. But if we enter a very deep level of consciousness, we will perceive reality differently. Mystics and great masters, who have achieved very deep levels of consciousness through meditation, report that nothing is discontinuous, that everything is harmoniously united in a continuous exchange of energy. Hence, everything in the universe is interrelated and interdependent. There is truth in the poetic saying that the fall of a sparrow is felt at the most distant star.

Leonardo da Vinci was not only a great painter and sculptor, but also a great scientist, engineer, inventor and visionary. How and where did he get his unending flow of inspiration and creative ideas? Through meditation, from the Universal Mind. He would often stare nonchalantly into a heap of ashes, and enter a state of deep meditation. Beautiful ideas would then appear to his subconscious mind.

Mozart would go on long coach rides to the countryside. There, in a meditative state of mind, he would hear beautiful music in his subconscious mind. Thomas Edison said that his inventions came to him through the infinite forces in the universe, and he received them while in a relaxed, meditative mood.

One of my best disciples, who has helped me tremendously in spreading the message of Shaolin Chi Kung and kungfu, is Ng Kowi Beng. He was an engineer in a factory, and although he was grossly underpaid, he worked diligently and ungrudgingly. I told him to meditate and contact the Universal Mind to help him build a factory of his own. At that time there appeared to be no way that he could build his own factory. But Kowi Beng had confidence in me and practiced what I had taught him. One of my happiest moments was when he told me, a few months later, that he was going to start a factory. Now he is a successful manufacturer.

How does the subconscious mind in meditation give us inspiration and enhance our creativity? It is like a superb computer. Not only does it store all our knowledge and experience, it also has access to the infinite wisdom and intelligence of the Universal Mind.

### Reaching the Subconscious Mind in Meditation

First you should focus your mind in meditation. Sit cross-legged in a quiet place. You may use the double lotus position, with both your soles facing up; the single lotus position, with only one sole facing up, as in *figure 17.1*; or an ordinary cross- legged position, with neither sole facing up. Place a hard pillow under your buttocks if necessary. Place your hands gently on your knees.

If you find these positions difficult, just sit upright on a chair with your palms on your thighs and your feet firmly on the floor, as in *figure 17.2*.

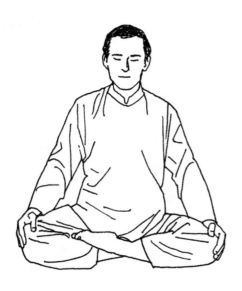

*Fig. 17.1 The Single Lotus Position—Lohan Style*

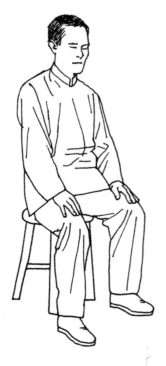

*Fig. 17.2 Sitting Upright for Meditation*

Close your eyes and breathe naturally. Clear your mind of all thoughts. Then visualize a round spot, like the golden sun or the silvery moon, in your mind. Try to keep the vision of this spot in your mind as long as possible. Do not worry if the spot changes color.

Various thoughts will start appearing in your mind. As soon as a thought appears, gently throw it out, and keep visualizing your round spot. It will be difficult at first, and you may visualize the spot for only one or two seconds. But if you practice regularly, you will increase the time of focus.

Initially practice this meditation for about five minutes. During that time you will see and lose the spot numerous times. Gradually you will be able to see the spot in your mind for longer and longer periods. Do not be discouraged at the difficulty. Indeed, if you can focus your mind on the spot for thirty seconds at a time, you will have achieved a lot. As you progress you can increase the time for each meditation; but it is the quality of the focusing of your mind, rather than the length of time you sit cross-legged, that is important. Complete the meditation by rubbing your palms together to warm your eyes, and massaging your face and legs. Then briskly walk about thirty paces.

Practice this mind-focusing meditation daily for at least four months. By that time you should be able to focus your mind on the spot quite well. You should also feel inner peace. Then you will be able to use your meditative skill to enhance your insight, inspiration, and creativity to solve problems or for a variety of other purposes. This is how to do it.

Sit cross-legged or upright on a chair, and go into meditation. When you have reached your subconscious level—when you appear to be unaware of, or not bothered by your immediate surrounding—gently but firmly meditate on your particular work or project. You may fix your mind on only one aspect of your work, such as a painting you might be working on, or review a whole process, such as the various stages of a scientific research project. If relevant images flash into your mental vision, do not ask questions, but just serenely take note of them. At this subconscious level, where you are linked to the Universal Mind, you are not merely imagining your work or project, but seeing it in the full glory of celestial light. Fresh insight, inspiration, or creativity may flash across your mind then, or may surface later when you are relaxing.

Alternatively, for more prosaic uses, you can pose a problem and await an answer from your subconscious. You need to frame your question before you meditate, so that when you are at the subconscious level, you can ask the question unhesitatingly and confidently. You should ask only one thing at a time, and you must be very specific about what you ask. For example, do not just ask, "Give me some insight to help me with my marketing." Instead, say something like, "My

company has come out with this new product, a talking computer. Show me the best way I can market it so as to bring the most benefits to my customers, my company and myself."

You should repeat your request or question over many meditations. Although your subconscious may occasionally flash you an answer immediately, generally it needs time to amass the necessary information from the Universal Mind, assess various possibilities, and then provide you with the best solution. The solution may come to you during meditation or in your normal waking hours when you are relaxed and least expecting it; and it may be revealed to you symbolically. Sometimes you may think the response odd, but it will almost always turn out to be the best solution.

Your subconscious mind is a very powerful tool. It must never be abused. If you use it for evil means, it will inevitably bring you harm. This is not some moralizing platitude to deter would-be wrongdoers; it is a statement of universal truth. We become what we think.

# CHAPTER EIGHTEEN

# Chi Kung Feats You Will Not Believe

What things soever ye desire, when ye pray believe that ye receive
them, and ye shall have them.

Mark 11:24

## Some Incredible Chi Kung Feats

Would you believe it if someone told you that Chi Kung masters could pass *chi* through walls, causing people in another room to sway involuntarily; could energize water which healed patients who drank it; could see through someone's skin and muscles into his organs; could disperse clouds and stop rain; could project their minds or travel astrally to distant places; could recall past lives; or could communicate with higher intelligence? Few people are inclined to believe such feats. Some might attack such claims as quackery. Years ago, I myself would have thought them crazy. But now I know that they are true because my senior students and I have performed all these feats!

Even if I provide proofs and demonstrations, many, even among those who witness them, still say that such feats are impossible and that what they have seen is either some kind of coincidence, or has been faked. One of the features of human nature is that we find it difficult to believe anything which does not conform to conventional wisdom, no matter how convincing the evidence.

Why, then, are these fantastic feats described here? The answer is: to make the book complete, for these feats constitute an important, though arcane, aspect of the fascinating art of Chi Kung. If you really do not want to believe in such "nonsense," you are welcome to remain skeptical. But I hope that some enterprising minds will find in these descriptions valuable information that may open up some exciting knowledge that can benefit mankind.

## How Societies Treated Brave Pioneers

Before examining these incredible feats, it is illuminating, albeit shocking, to discover how society has in the past reacted to great men and women who courageously announced revolutionary ideas that later proved to be true. When Galileo, in the seventeenth century, suggested that the earth was not the center of the universe, he was imprisoned for life. In the next century, when Lavoisier, the father of modern chemistry, said that air and water were compounds, he was ridiculed and reminded that air, water, fire and earth had been accepted as elements for centuries. In the nineteenth century, when George Stephenson proposed the building of railway lines, he was confronted with suggestions that locomotives would set houses on fire and the noise would drive people mad.[11]

Responses to medical breakthroughs were equally stubborn, even cruel. In the Middle Ages, Pierre Brissot was rewarded for his protests against excessive bloodletting by being ostracized; he died in exile. When Michael Servetus suggested the idea of pulmonary circulation, he was burnt to death as a heretic.

As late as the nineteenth century, when Semmelweis discovered that if surgeons washed their hands with chlorine solution they vastly reduced the mortality rate on the operation table, he was so severely abused by his colleagues that he became mad and died in an asylum. In 1829, when Jules Cloquet reported to his medical academy that he had successfully used mesmerism to operate on an elderly woman without causing her any pain, the academy was naive enough to reply that the patient must have pretended to feel no pain! In 1843, when John Elliotson, considered as one of the most brilliant doctors in his country, published case histories of his successful use of mesmerism to deaden pain in surgical operations, he was ordered to stop the practice in his own hospital, which he helped to found. Elliotson resigned and made one of the most inspiring statements I have ever read:

> The Institution was established for the discovery and dissemination of truth. We should lead the public, not the public us. All other considerations are secondary. The sole question is whether the matter is the truth or not.[12]

These are only some of the many examples of society's reactions to new discoveries and unconventional ideas. With the understanding, therefore, that today's bizarre theories may be tomorrow's norms, let us examine the following Chi Kung feats with an open mind.

## Channeling Chi through a Wall

In 1989, the Moral Uplifting Society in Taiping, Malaysia invited me to give a talk on Chi Kung and demonstrate some feats. My student, Leong, went into a room, with side windows that were left open so that the spectators could see his performance. About twenty volunteers, whom Leong had not met before, stood in two lines in a hall, separated from Leong by a brick wall. They and Leong could not see each other. Leong waved his hands about to transmit *chi* through the wall to the volunteers. About a minute later the volunteers started to sway involuntarily. Soon some of them were moving vigorously; others were performing some sort of graceful involuntary dances. Roughly six hundred members of the public witnessed this demonstration.

The explanation of this phenomenon is simple. Leong's *chi* passed through the wall to the volunteers and moved the *chi* inside their bodies. Since they were relaxed and co-operative, their own *chi* caused their bodies to sway and move.

A similar experiment was performed by a Chi Kung master in China some years ago for a team of American scientists who were investigating the working of *chi*. When the scientists asked the master to stop sending *chi*, the volunteers in the other room continued to move. The scientists asked the master to control the volunteers and stop their movements, but the master said he could not because their *chi* was still flowing and would continue to do so for some time.

The scientists therefore said that the exercise was fraudulent because the experimenter had no objective control over his experiment. Since the volunteers' movements were caused by the master's *chi*, the scientists expected the master to be able to start and stop their movements at will.

## Helpful Guidelines for Researchers

This experiment illustrates a few important points that may be useful to researchers. First, there was a communication gap: neither side was clear about what the other wanted. Secondly, it was unfair for the scientists to impose their terms on a situation where those terms would not be appropriate. Perhaps the scientists felt that their rigid scientific investigative methods were the best, and any experiments that could not be measured in their terms could not qualify as scientific or valid. What they did not realize, or refused to accept, was that these terms might not apply to Chi Kung, which uses a totally different paradigm—in the same way that if the Chinese were to use their principles of *yin-yang* and the *Five Elemental Processes* as a yardstick, many routine scientific experiments might not "work." It is reasonable to expect that someone who wants to know about Chi Kung should at least listen to what a Chi Kung master has to say, and then test him on his terms of reference.

Thirdly, there was a conflict of attitudes. The scientists thought they were helping the Chi Kung master, providing him with an opportunity to elevate his art to the status of science. If they had been mean-spirited, they might even have done everything in their power to discredit the master, irrespective of the evidence.[13] On the other hand, the master likely felt that he was doing the foreigners a favor, sharing with them secret information which he might not even have told his neighbors. He would not care a hoot whether his art was labeled scientific or otherwise; after all, it had worked for him and other people for centuries.

## Energizing Water for Therapy

Zainab was about six years old when her father carried her into our Chi Kung clinic. For the previous two years she had not been able to walk. My senior disciple, Chan Chee Kong, who is a consultant engineer by profession but gives Chi Kung therapy in his spare time because of his care for others, attended to her. He found that Zainab's *chi* flow was weak and was blocked at a number of points at her legs. He opened many of her energy points and channeled *chi* to her. But a major problem was that, like most children, she could not keep still, making the transmission of *chi* to specific points difficult. I suggested to Chan that he transmit *chi* to a glass of water, and let her drink it. After about four months of drinking this energized water every alternate day, coupled with Chi Kung massage and induced *chi* flow exercises, Zainab could walk reasonably well.

Scientists in China have discovered that water energized by Chi Kung masters has a different molecular structure than ordinary water, but that it returns to normal after a few days. I wonder whether the energized water helps to correct the disturbed DNA structure of a sick person, thereby making him well.

When I was young, I always marveled at the way in which patients were cured of their illnesses by consecrated water. In Chinese society (and other Eastern societies), patients often consult spiritual healers when conventional and other medicines cannot heal them. The spiritual healer goes into a trance, communicates with a god or higher intelligence, and then writes some magic formula on yellow papers. These talismans are burned and the ashes mixed in water to be drunk by the patients.

The question here is not whether this is mere superstition, but whether it works. Generally it does. I am convinced that its success is not due to psychological or placebo effects. I believe that divine energy is transmitted to the water via the yellow talismans. Similarly, when holy men of various religions bless their followers, divine energy is transmitted to them. Perhaps it was divine energy, as well as faith, that enabled healing by holy men and women to be one of the main healing systems in the West for more than ten centuries.

This theory assumes the presence of higher beings. My master, Sifu Ho Fatt Nam, used to warn people not to do evil, as higher beings, whom the Chinese refer to as gods, are all around us. It is interesting to note that modern Westerners are the only people in the history of mankind who do not believe in higher beings. These higher beings, like everything else, including ourselves, are forms of energy.

### Seeing through Your Body into Your Organs

Many years ago when my son, Wong Chun Nga, told me he had seen three phalanges inside his friend's finger, I was curious, for it was not common for a boy of ten to know that sort of thing. Later he told me he could sometimes see people's internal organs. When I asked him to see my internal organs, he said he couldn't because they were well protected by *chi*. Then I tested him by focusing my *chi* at various energy fields, or by channeling it to various parts of the body. He could tell me just where my *chi* was concentrated. One evening after I had completed my Chi Kung training, my son said that he could see a lot of dog's fur flowing into my body. I could not see any fur around me, but then I realized that it was cosmic energy that my son could see, which he mistook for dog's fur!

One night, my son said he could see green energy flowing out from my meditation room on to the telephone wires and along the wires for some time before it disappeared into the sky. Another night he saw energy shooting up from the room, through the ceiling, very high into the sky, and then bursting out like fireworks in many directions. He even psychically heard a soft explosion as the energy burst out. On both these nights I was experimenting with distant chi transmission (which will be described in the next chapter).

My son's psychic sight is a very useful skill (which I do not have) for diagnosis. He could accurately tell which internal organs were injured, as they were surrounded by dark-colored *chi*. As I transmitted my *chi* to patients to cure their injuries, he could see a ray of bright greenish-yellow light flowing from my fingers into the patients and dispersing the dark-colored *chi*.

I can think of two possible explanations for my son's psychic sight. First, the electromagnetic spectrum known to science today extends from wavelengths of 0.000000047 microns to over 30 kilometers; but the range of wavelengths our normal eyes can see is extremely small—from 0.4 to 0.8 microns (0.0004-0.0008 millimeters)! By practicing Chi Kung, perhaps one may expand this very limited range and so be able to see some things that ordinary people cannot.

Secondly, our eyes, like the rest of our physical bodies, are only agents of our minds. Actually, we see with our minds, not with our eyes. In my son's case, it is possible that Chi Kung practice has improved his mind so that he can perceive what normal eyes cannot see. Indeed he told me that on those occasions when he could not see clearly, he focused his mind and the vision flashed across into him.

### Dispersing Clouds in the Sky

At 5 PM on September 21, 1989 hundreds of people waited in front of the Taiping Moral Uplifting Society to witness a public demonstration: my disciple Cheng Shang Shou and I were to disperse clouds in the sky.

First I focused my energy at my abdominal energy field, held my index finger and middle finger together by hooking the other two fingers with my thumb in a hand form called Sword Fingers, and aimed them at the center of a cloud in the sky. Using concentrated mind power, I

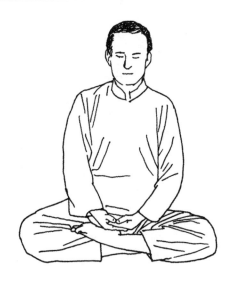

*Fig. 18.1 The Single Lotus Position - Buddha Style*

Sit cross-legged, or upright on a chair. It is important that your head is tilted slightly, and your spine is straight. If you sit cross-legged, place your palms on your knees as in the previous meditation, or in front of you on your legs, as in *figure 18.1*, with one palm on top of the other and the thumbs slightly touching.

Gently close your eyes and clear your mind of all thoughts. Breathe naturally and then forget about your breathing. Keep your mind empty. As soon as any thought enters your mind, gently but firmly throw it out. Meditate on the void or emptiness for about five minutes, and experience its joyous tranquility. Try to keep your body generally still, although some slight movement is permissible.

Gradually increase your meditation time to about fifteen minutes as you progress. In our school of Chi Kung, which is called Shaolin Cosmos Chi Kung, we prefer quality to quantity. If you can sit cross-legged for five minutes and have a total of two minutes' meditation on the void (or on one point, as in the previous chapter), you will have done admirably. This is better than sitting for half an hour, with fleeting moments of void or one-pointedness hardly adding up to a minute, but with twenty-nine minutes of mental chaos. You may use this "void-type" meditation (like the "one-pointed type") for enhancing insight, inspiration and creativity, for solving problems, and for other wholesome purposes. It is advisable to have a master to supervise you in meditation practice.

If you practice consistently, you may have strange sensations, like feeling as if you have lost part or whole of your physical body, or as if you have expanded enormously. These are natural developments. But if you feel mentally uncomfortable, frightened, oppressed, or any similar unpleasant sensations, you should stop practicing, at least temporarily.

The mind is the most powerful tool in the world. Give it the respect it deserves by using it for wholesome purposes only.

channeled my chi to the cloud. Then I moved my fingers round and round to "cut" the cloud into pieces. Soon the cloud dispersed, watched by hundreds of spectators. Next, Cheng Shang Shou repeated the performance.

This public demonstration was reported in the *Guang Min Daily News* on September 27, 1989, and in great detail in the *Mau Sang News* on October 7, 1989.

### Experiencing Joyous Tranquility

Meditation is necessary for all of these amazing feats. There are numerous techniques, but they can be classified into two main types. Citing Joseph Goldstein, Daniel Goleman supplies an apt and interesting guide:

It's simple mathematics, he said. All meditation systems either aim for One or Zero—union with God or emptiness. The path to the One is through concentration on Him, to the Zero is insight into the voidness of one's mind.[14]

Having aimed at One in the previous meditation exercise (see Chapter 17), let us now aim at Zero.

# CHAPTER NINETEEN

# *Distant Chi Transmission*

> No one who puts forward a new theory has any claim to be embraced, kissed and congratulated, but the very least he can reasonably expect is, that his theory will be seriously examined and discussed.
>
> Erich von Daniken

### Can Energy Be Transmitted by Man over a Great Distance?

In 1988 I caused a huge public controversy when I made an announcement that was carried in all major Chinese and English language newspapers. I said that Chi Kung masters could transmit chi over great distances to cure illnesses.

As I knew full well that few people would believe me, I announced that I was ready to be tested, stressing that it was not a challenge, but a sincere attempt to share useful knowledge that was already known in ancient times. I also appealed to other Chi Kung masters to work together to develop this art further for the benefit of humanity.

The response was tremendous—and negative! There was a concerted, unrelenting attempt to deride and mock me; and my attackers found my suggestion so outlandish that none thought it necessary to test my claim before debunking it. Nevertheless, I suppose I was lucky not to be burned at the stake, as might have happened in the past.

### A Public Experiment on Distant Chi Transmission

Instead of arguing with my opponents, I chose to show the validity of my statement by means of a public experiment. In February 1989, after the initial fury had died down, the Malaysian national Chinese newspaper, *Shin Min Daily News*, sponsored an open test spread over one month. Volunteers all over the country were invited to be recipients of *chi* transmitted from a distance.

In the experiment, I was to transmit *chi*—from Sungai Petani to Kuala Lumpur, a distance of about five hundred kilometers; and on different days my senior disciple, Chan Chee Kong, was to transmit *chi* from Kuala Lumpur to Sungai Petani. The people to receive *chi* were selected by the *Shin Min Daily News* from applicants who responded to their open invitation. Except for one person, all the recipients selected were unknown to Chan Chee Kong and me.

Besides transmitting *chi* to one person at a time, I also transmitted it to a group of six recipients. Pressmen and independent witnesses were present at both the transmitting and the receiving stations, and they communicated with each other or with the recipients over the telephone immediately after the *chi* transmissions, to compare notes and check results.

The results were overwhelming, with a success rate of ninety-five percent, higher than our average of eighty percent during normal practice. The experiment was published as headline news in many newspapers, including the *Sin Min Daily News* (19 February, and 9, 17 and 21 March 1989), the *Nanyang Commercial Press* (14 and 19 March 1989), the *New Night News* (16 March 1989), the *New Straits Times* (10 and 17 March 1989), the *Star* (21 March 1989), the *Mun Sang News* (1 April 1989) and the *United Post* (25 April 1989).

### What the Recipients Said about the Transmission

The following are some quotations from the statements of recipients, describing their experiences in the public experiment.

1. **Goh, male, aged 37, businessman.** "At first I resisted, but as the chi became stronger and stronger, I cooperated. The chi moved my body. I swayed forward and backward, left and right, and I felt warm."
2. **Chen, female, businesswoman.** "I had no Chi Kung training. My breathing became fast, and my body began to vibrate. Even my joints emitted some sound. At first I thought all this was something from the Arabian Nights, but now I'm convinced that distant chi transmission is possible."
3. **Ti, female, aged 19, painter.** "Chi entered through my head and face. I felt as though there was a breeze around me, like I was floating or on top of a mountain. I did not move of my own volition."
4. **Major Tee, male, aged 43, army officer.**

"Congratulations, Mr. Wong. Your chi was very powerful. I felt it flowing into my body. I've never felt like this before. It was very pleasant, and I am now full of power. I can testify that distant chi transmission is a reality."
5. **Lee, female, aged 37, housewife.** "Thank you, Sifu Wong, for your wonderful chi transmission. I've done chi flow exercises previously, but I've never felt like this before. I moved vigorously, and I started to hit and massage my own body. I danced gracefully."
6. **Tan, male, aged 35, teacher.** "I practice Chi Kung too, but it is different from Mr. Wong's style. I have read about distant chi transmission, and I believe it is true. So this was a golden opportunity for me to experience it myself. The chi flowed round my body. I began to vibrate and move involuntarily, but it was very comfortable."

One interesting aspect was that both Chan and I could tell how the recipients moved. We described their movements to the witnesses, who immediately telephoned the recipients and found our descriptions generally right. We could do this, firstly, because by the way in which we transmitted *chi*, we had some influence over the recipients' movements; and secondly because we saw their movements in our meditation during the transmission process.

### Four Fundamental Concepts about Chi

Distant *chi* transmission is a reality, though it is hard for most people to believe—just as it is hard for those not familiar with particle physics to believe that the experimenter's thoughts actually influence the result of his experiment.

To understand how *chi* can be transmitted over great distances, it is necessary to understand the following basic concepts. They are not new, nor are they restricted to the field of Chi Kung. They have been discussed and accepted by Chi Kung masters as well as Confucian scholars, Taoist priests, Buddhist monks, military strategists, martial artists, men of literature, politicians, physicians, philosophers and scientists throughout Chinese history. The four concepts are:

1.  *Chi* is energy.
2.  *Chi* has material reality.
3.  *Chi* is the basic element of which everything in the universe is constituted.
4.  *Chi* fills the whole universe and hence is a universal medium.

### Chi as Energy and with Material Reality

The concept of *chi* as energy has been amply illustrated in Chinese records since ancient times. Its meaning is very wide, ranging from natural and mental energy to life and spiritual energy. Po Yang Fu, more than 2500 years ago, described the cause of earthquakes as the disharmony of sky and earth energy. The great strategist, Sun Tzu, counseled that an army should avoid the vibrant energy of the enemy in the morning, and attack his restful energy at night. Zao Bi, a famous man of letters, said that *chi* is the primary factor in great literature. Hence there are different kinds of *chi*. In Chi Kung, it usually refers to vital or life energy when it is inside the body, and to cosmic energy when it is outside.

As *chi* is intangible and invisible (to ordinary people), many fail to realize that it is material and real. Some people even think that it is simply a product of the imagination. But now, researchers in China, using modern scientific apparatus, have discovered that the *chi* transmitted by Chi Kung masters consists of infrared rays, static electricity, electromagnetic waves, subsonic waves, and certain particle flows. Li Zhao Hui and Huo Xin

Chang startled scientific circles with their discovery that it also consists of impulses or messages that can be transmitted from the mind of a Chi Kung master, and these impulses affect the size, weight, and growth rate of cultured microorganisms.[15] Modern physics has revealed that energy and matter are two aspects of the same reality, and that they constantly change from one into the other. Chi Kung masters and Chinese philosophers have known this for a long time.

For a long time we thought that the atom was the smallest unit of matter, but now scientists have shown that the atom can be broken down into the neutron, the proton and the electron. If we think of an atom as a circle ten meters in diameter, the nucleus (neutrons and proton) would not be bigger than one millimeter in the center, with the electrons, 1840 times less massive, whirling around at the edge of the circle. This picture provides us with some idea of the immense void that exists in an atom. Scientists are still not certain what is actually in this void, although most believe that it is a continuous spread of energy, and that subatomic particles are merely concentrations of energy. Chi Kung masters and Chinese philosophers since ancient times have stressed that *chi* or energy is the basic stuff of the universe, and that the negative, positive and neutral aspects of energy—known in classical Chinese as *yin*, *yang* and *zhong chi*—continuously integrate and disintegrate to form and break up matter.

### The Constituent and Medium of the Universe

*Chi* fills the whole universe; in fact, the universe is *chi*. Cheng Yi Shan summarizes ancient Chinese thinking on *chi* and the universe in these words:

> All things, including all the landforms, oceans and living things on earth, the earth itself and all heavenly bodies....are the products of changing

states of *chi*. The current universe is a state in the endless progression of changing *chi*. This changing *chi* has its definite principles, order and laws. The cause of this changing *chi* is its intrinsic nature of opposing yet complementary *yin-yang*. [16]

As *chi* permeates the universe, it also acts as a universal medium. The ancient Chinese used this concept to explain many natural phenomena that puzzled the ordinary people, such as the attraction of iron by magnets, the influence of the moon on tides, and the rhythmic life cycles of invertebrates. For example, although the sea is separated from the moon by a great distance, the moon's influence on the tides is possible because the intervening *chi* acts as a connecting medium.

Man, like all other things, is permeated by *chi* and united with the universe, which is also permeated by *chi*. This is the principle of cosmos-man unity, an important concept in advanced Chi Kung. The romantic Taoist sage, Chuang Tzu (Zhuang Zi in romanized Chinese), said:

The cosmos and I live on forever.
All things and I are united as one.

Wei Nan Tzu explained that all things are connected by *chi*, and when the *chi* of one thing or event mingles with the *chi* of another, both will be affected. In this way, the deep compassion and sincerity of great men can move heaven and earth. This perhaps explains why information learned by creatures in one part of the world seems to benefit similar creatures in other parts of the world, although there is no visible contact between them—an exciting discovery that has puzzled modern biologists.

### The Theory of Distant Chi Transmission

As *chi* is a universal medium that connects all things, a Chi Kung master can use it to transmit his *chi*-impulses to another person a great distance away. This is shown in *figure 19.1*, where *M* is the Chi Kung master, and *R1* and *R2* are recipients.

*M* and *R1* are connected by a band of *chi*, *AB*. Impulses from *M* can be transmitted along this band to *R1*. Similarly, impulses from *M* can be transmitted to *R2* along the band *CD*. As chi is a form of energy, it can pass through any obstacles between the master and the recipients.

Let us imagine that *AB* and *CD* are solid rods.

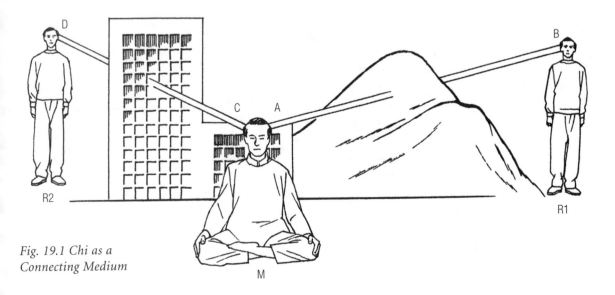

*Fig. 19.1 Chi as a Connecting Medium*

If we push at *A* and at *C* at the same time, both *R1* and *R2* will instantly feel the push at *B* and at *D*. Hence, although *R1* and *R2* are at different distances from *M*, they will receive *chi* the instant the master transmits it.

Two essential questions arise: how do we use the intervening *chi* as a connecting medium, and how do we transmit *chi*-impulses along this medium?

The answer to the first is that we merge the *chi* in the body with the *chi* of the universe, that is, we achieve cosmos-man unity.

The body, like the space around it, is made up of atoms, which are electrons spinning round nuclei. The latest discoveries in physics show that electrons, protons and neutrons are not so much solid particles as clouds of differently charged electricity—a concept propounded by masters of various great ancient civilizations long ago. In other words, our bodies, the surrounding atmosphere, and everything else are a continuous spread of energy, with concentrations that we conveniently call particles. Because our eyes are grossly inadequate, we do not see this continuity of undifferentiated energy, but see its gross concentrations as differentiated entities.

We see the body as a separate unit from its surroundings, with the skin as the boundary. But at the subatomic level—where physicists with their elaborate, fine instruments, and mystics in deep meditation can reach—there is no boundary. The particles at the edge of one concentration (in this case, the body) merely thin out and merge with the particles of the surrounding air. We actually cannot tell where the body ends and the surrounding air begins. When we experience this reality—rather than just knowing about it—we attain cosmos-man unity.

There is a poetic Chi Kung term to describe this reality: man in energy, energy in man. It means that we exist in a sea of energy that surrounds us (our universe is energy); and at the same time there is a sea of energy inside us (we are made of

energy). A rough analogy is as follows. Imagine we have a cube of ice with an open hollow in the center, making it like a bowl. Fill this ice bowl with water, and submerge it in a huge tank of water. After a while we cannot tell the difference between the water in the bowl and the water in the tank. When the ice melts, everything in the tank becomes one undifferentiated unity.

As to how we transmit *chi*-impulses along the medium, the *chi* that a master transmits to a distant recipient is different from the *chi* he transmits to someone in front of him. When the recipient is in front of him, the *chi* transmitted is physical: it comes from the master's *chi* and travels through his palms, fingers or any part of his body directly into the recipient, as shown in *figure 19.2*.

If the recipient is very far away, it is not feasible to send physical *chi* directly. The master has to transform his *chi* into *shen* or mind-power, and then transmit this *shen* to the distant recipient, as in *figure 19.3*.

Mind-power is transmitted in the form of impulses. The master's impulses strike one end of the *chi*-medium, and are transmitted by the medium to the other end. When the impulses reach the recipient at the other end, he receives the impulses as *chi*. But this *chi* is not the same as the *chi* that comes physically from the master,

*Fig. 19.2 Transmitting Chi Directly*

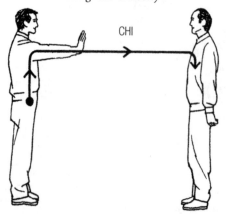

CHI

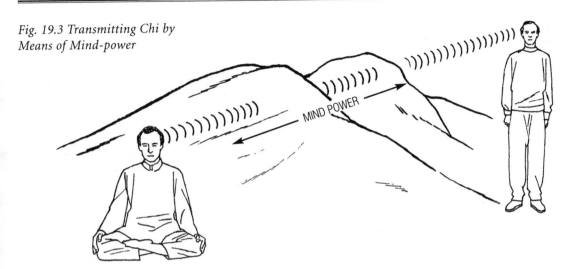

*Fig. 19.3 Transmitting Chi by Means of Mind-power*

although it is similar—in the same way that the voice you hear over the telephone is not actually the caller's voice, although they are similar.

Hence, distant *chi* transmission requires the attainment of two higher levels of Chi Kung training; transforming *chi* into *shen* and merging the mind with the cosmos.

### The Art of Wisdom

The following meditation exercise, known as the *Art of Wisdom,* will help you to merge with the cosmos. It was introduced by the famous master of *Chanmizhong* Chi Kung, Liu Han Wen, who generously revealed what was once a closely-guarded secret.

The *Art of Wisdom* can be performed while standing, or while sitting on a chair or cross-legged. However, it is best to start with the standing posture; the sitting posture is for more advanced practitioners. As you would expect, the uninitiated may find some steps peculiar or puzzling.

1. Stand upright with your arms hanging loosely at your sides.

2. Close your eyes and relax.

3. Think of opening the *huiyin* energy point (at the anus).

4. Starting from the fingers and toes, slightly move or vibrate the whole body, until your spine and your internal organs and tissues are in gentle motion induced by internal *chi* movements. (Those who can perform *Induced Chi Flow*, as explained in Chapter 4, will be better able to follow this step.) See these motions in your mind's eye, and listen to the sound of your muscles and joints loosening.

5. Breathe naturally. Be aware that every tissue and cell of your body is breathing. Your breathing will become so natural that you will soon forget about it. Feel joyful at your heart. Let this joy radiate throughout your body.

6. With your normal eyes still closed, open your third (or psychic) eye. Through your third eye, visualize some natural majestic scene, like a gigantic waterfall or the great expanse of the sky. Imagine that your body covering, your hair and skin, is expanded and dispersed into the vast universe, and your mind is merged with the infinite cosmos.

7. Reverse the visualization, from the vast

expanse of the universe to focus on your abdomen as the center.

8. Next (or in another session) stand with your arms open in front and above you, as in *figure 19.4*.

9. Think of your *baihui* energy point (at the crown of your head) being open, and stand firmly, as if rooted to the ground.

10. Think of your two *yongquan* energy points (at the soles of your feet) being open.

11. Visualize cosmic energy flowing from high up in the sky and entering you at your *baihui*, palms and shoulders, flowing through your body, cleansing and energizing you, and exiting from your *huiyin* and *yongquan* deep into the earth. Visualize this harmonious flow of cosmic energy linking heaven, man (you) and earth.

12. Reverse the process, visualizing good earth energy flowing through you to the sky.

13. Repeat these downward and upward flows of energy a few times.

14. Bring your palms together above your head, and lower them to chest level as if in prayer (see *figure 19.5*).

15. Let your mind expand to the infinite and merge with the universe, attaining cosmos-man unity. Your breathing will no longer be at your direction; it will become a function of the universe. As you naturally breathe in, your abdomen is the center of the universe, drawing cosmic energy from the furthest reach of the infinite; and as you breathe out, your life energy affects the furthest reach of the cosmos. You pulsate with the universe.

16. To complete the exercise, lower your palms and place them one on top of the other at your qihai energy field at your abdomen (about two inches below the navel). With your eyes still closed, look inwardly (or psychically) at your inside. Feel the pearl of energy at your abdomen. Then rub your

palms, warm your eyes with them, open your eyes, and walk about briskly.

If you practice this *Art of Wisdom* conscientiously, do not be surprised to find psychic or supernormal powers developing. It is easy for humans, in their numerous moments of weakness, to abuse such powers, which are almost sacred. We must constantly guard against this abuse—for our own sake.

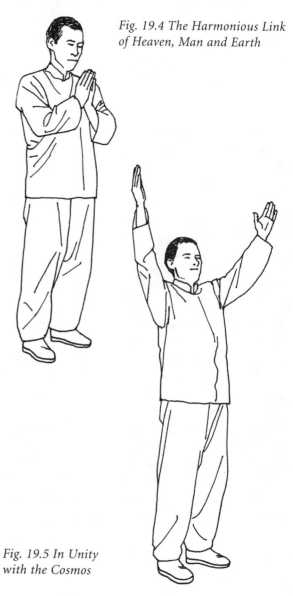

*Fig. 19.4 The Harmonious Link of Heaven, Man and Earth*

*Fig. 19.5 In Unity with the Cosmos*

# PART SIX

# The Supreme Achievement of Chi Kung

# CHAPTER TWENTY

# A Conceptual Framework to Explain Miracles

> For many years investigations on telepathy and other phenomena of extrasensory perception have taken place, but no genius has appeared who can make the necessary speculations which will make these things cease to be mysterious and unexpected and fall into order.
>
> Robert H. Thouless

## Scientific Study of Miracles

As Dr. Thouless (who has given us a wonderful book, *Straight and Crooked Thinking*) is a psychologist who believes in objective, quantitative facts, and not a mystic or a spiritual teacher who ventures into the "supernatural," it is understandable that he is not aware of the numerous speculations and explanations, not only of extrasensory perception (ESP) but also of the more incredible phenomena that we call miracles. But what is "supernatural?" Watson answers succinctly:

> There is, when you look at it closely, no such thing as the supernatural. All we have are reports of experiences which seem to be beyond natural explanation—but we do have these in astonishing abundance. And the reports have become so frequent and so widespread that they are very difficult for anyone with real scientific curiosity to ignore. [17]

It was not until the 1930s, when Dr. Rhine, the father of modern parapsychology, made the study of psi a respectable discipline by using strict scientific procedures, and discovered that at least one out of five people possess some ESP abilities, that the (Western) public in general felt comfortable discussing psychic powers.

But it is doubtful whether the scientific method, as normally practiced with its insistence on objectivity, quantification and repeatability, is suitable for testing or understanding ESP and other miracles. Miraculous events are, by nature, subjective, qualitative, and singular. For example, if you read what is in your friend's mind at any given moment and he confirms it, there are no objective ways (other than his confirmation) to prove the validity of your claim. An experimenter could, of course, supply a specific subject for your friend to think about, but then you might not be able to read thoughts at that particular time. Moreover, there is no satisfactory way to quantify how accurately you read his mind, because this particular telepathic experience is singular and not repeatable, and even the telepathic skill itself may not easily be repeated, unless you are a master.

This does not mean that we cannot study miracles scientifically. But if any study or test is to be meaningful, the scientists, without relinquishing their strict control, must also be able to view the experiment from the subjects' perspective. This includes some basic understanding of why and how miracles happen, and a willingness to assess the miracles according to the terms of reference commonly used by miracle performers themselves.

### Miracles Have Happened and Are Happening

Miracles are so called because they seem to be beyond the laws of nature as conventional scientists and ordinary people know them. Miracles are a reality; they have happened, not only as recorded in responsible texts from the past, but also in reality today. Many of the things that my disciples and I have done—like telepathy, clairvoyance, astral traveling, distant healing, dispersing clouds and stopping rain—are termed miracles by ordinary people, although we stress that they can all be explained by natural laws, and can be done by anyone who has put in sufficient effort to acquire the art.

Many of the miracles demonstrated by great Chi Kung masters in China today defy belief. In May 1986, the Taoist Chi Kung master Wang Li Ping used his mental impulses to summon hundreds of squirrels from the neighborhood to gather at a Chi Kung training center in a Beijing suburb. Zhang Bao Sheng, who is called "the foremost psychic in China," could transport the shoe you are wearing to another place without you knowing it.[18]

Indian and Tibetan masters are well known for their miracles. It is widely acknowledged that holy ashes, which can be used for healing purposes, have materialized on photographs of the living saint, Sai Baba, in homes of his followers. The yogi Paramahansa Yogananda describes the materialization of a palace in the Himalayas by Mahavatara Babaji.[19] Tibetan monks travel over vast areas at tremendous speed, as though skimming the surface of the earth. They keep themselves warm during winter nights without external aid.[20]

Performing miracles, of course, is not the exclusive domain of Eastern Masters. The famous Polish psychic, Wolf Mersing, who was tested by Einstein, Freud, Gandhi and Stalin, could telepathically project his thought into other people to control or cloud their minds.[21] The great American psychic, Edgar Cayce, left over 14,000 documented psychic readings, presently available at the Association for Research and Enlightenment, Virginia, for public investigation.[22]

Although the actual number of miracles is substantial, they are understandably not as common as, say, motor accidents. Hence many people may not have seen any with their own eyes; that of course does not mean that they do not happen. When my own master, Sifu Ho Fatt Nam, first told me that his master, physically far away, could travel astrally to watch his students practice their art, or that his senior classmate could walk through walls, I found it hard to accept, although I had great respect and love for my master, and believed that he was telling the truth. Similarly, when I told my senior disciples that they could transmit *chi* over great distance, they could not believe it until they did it for themselves.

### What the Masters Have Said about Miracles

When asked about miracles, most people will inevitably say they are impossible. If they happen to witness one, they will exclaim that it cannot be explained.

But miracles can be explained, and the best people to go to for an explanation are not scientists or philosophers, but the masters who can perform them—although some of these masters are scientists and philosophers themselves.

Mersing constantly emphasizes that there is nothing supernatural or mysterious in his ability to read thoughts. He insists that telepathy is simply a matter of harnessing natural laws. "The time is coming when man will understand all these phenomena," he said. "There is nothing strange. Only what is not yet commonplace."[23]

Zhang Bao Sheng also says that his feats are nothing new. He stresses that all the methods to develop, and the principles to explain, his miracles are readily found in classical Chinese texts, especially in the *Yi Jing* (*Book of Change*), and the concepts of *yin-yang*, *Pakua* (*Bagua* or the Eight Trigrams), and *wu xing* (or the *Five Elemental Processes*).

Yogananda explains the law of miracles as follows:

> A yogi who through perfect meditation has merged his consciousness with the Creator perceives the cosmical essence as light (vibrations of life energy): to him there is no difference between the light rays composing water and the light rays composing land. Free from matter-consciousness, free from the three dimensions of space and the fourth dimension of time, a master transfers his body of light with equal ease over or through the light rays of earth, water, fire, and air. [24]

Classical Chi Kung texts are rich in explanations of miracles as well as providing guidance on performing them, although many readers might not understand the arcane knowledge or believe its validity even if they had access to these texts.

Buddhist Chi Kung classifies miracles into six main types. Miracles are possible when a master, in his deep meditation, is able to see reality as it really is, as an infinite void impregnated with infinite consciousness (or energy). Four steps are necessary in developing miraculous abilities: the intention to do so, gradual progress, one-pointedness, and intense visualization. There are two schools of thought regarding the acquisition of such powers. One school, found especially among the Mahayana Buddhists, believes that these miraculous abilities are best used to save people; the other school, found particularly among the Theravada Buddhists, believes that these powers act as a

hindrance to one's enlightenment.

Miraculous powers are a natural development of the Taoist saints, that is, those Taoist masters who have attained immortality, either still in their physical living body or as discarnate beings. Lesser practitioners, who abuse these powers as black magic, will inevitably suffer the intrinsic result of (not extrinsic punishment for) their evil karmic effect, in this life or in subsequent ones. Taoists generally do not aim for these powers; they acquire them as by-products of their spiritual training. These bowers are possible because the highly developed mind (*shen*) of a master is able to manipulate energy (*qi*) and essence (*jing*) according to his wishes. Meditation to train the mind is essential.

The above descriptions provide invaluable explanations as well as useful guidelines for attaining miraculous powers. Though they come from different philosophical backgrounds, they generally say the same thing. Basically, they explain that miracles are possible when the master's mind merges with the Universal Mind, and the essential process is meditation.

Yet for laymen or scientists not familiar with these philosophies, these explanations are still bewildering. How does attaining unity with the Universal Mind make it possible to perform miracles? How does meditation lead to a unity with the Universal Mind?

A technique for reaching the Universal Mind through meditation was explained in Chapter 17. In the following section a few examples are discussed to illustrate how unity with the Universal Mind enables a master to use cosmic energy for performing miracles.

### Explanation of Miracles

The conceptual framework used to explain distant *chi* transmission in the previous chapter is also very useful for explaining miracles. This framework proposes that *chi* is energy, that it has material reality, that it is the basic stuff of the universe, and that it is also a universal medium.

As the whole universe is permeated with energy, every person, object, and event is organically connected, though our naked eyes see them as separate. When a person thinks, he creates vibrations in the universal energy. A master whose mind has been united with the Universal Mind—the infinite spread of conscious energy—can pick up these vibrations and translate them back into thoughts. Hence the master is able to read another person's mind, or has telepathic powers.

Space and time are real to us at our ordinary or conscious level, but at the subatomic or subconscious level, they have no significance. Hence, the mind in a deeply meditative state transcends space and time. This means that the master can pick up vibrations of other minds or events that occur not only far away, but also in the past and the future. In other words, he has powers of clairvoyance, reading the past, and divination.

Reading the past may be acceptable, but telling the future? How can someone predict anything that has not even happened? Past, present, and future are convenient constructs, and are relative. Karmic causes that will result in events in the future already exist now or existed in the past. A highly developed mind can interpret these karmic vibrations. A rough analogy is someone walking down a long corridor towards your room. If your ears are sharp, you can predict from his footsteps that he will appear in a few minutes.

Let us now look at another class of miracles. How does a master project his mind to another place, or to another person? How is astral travel possible? Actually we all project our minds to other people without realizing it. When you think of someone deeply, or try to influence their opinion mentally, you are performing mind projection, as your thought vibrations are transmitted along the universal energy to reach him. Of course, if you are not well trained, your effect is slight, and is often cancelled out by other mental vibrations.

The mind is independent of the physical body, and therefore may be projected to places or people far away; and this is greatly facilitated when the individual mind is merged with the Universal Mind. But for most people, the individual mind is imprisoned in the physical body. When the master realizes this, and liberates his mind from the bodily prison, he can travel astrally.

Another class of miracles involves psychokinesis and materialization. You have actually performed psychokinesis and materialization in many of the Chi Kung exercises described in this book. For example, when you visualize *chi* flowing to and from your abdomen in *Abdominal Breathing* (Chapter 6), you are practicing psychokinesis. When you visualize a pearl of *chi* forming at your abdomen in the *Gentle Small Universe* (Chapter 15), you are practicing materialization.

Of course, it is much easier to use your mind to direct your *chi* flow than psychically to transport your friend's shoe; easier to build a pearl of *chi* than to materialize a palace. But the principle is similar, except that in your case your sphere of operation is your own body, which is a small cosmos; whereas the master, after merging his mind with the Universal Mind, is operating the big cosmos like his body. Theoretically, if you know how to use a pound to buy bread, you also know how to use a million pounds to buy a castle, even though the amount, of course, is vastly different. Similarly, both materializing a pearl of chi and materializing a palace involve using mind to shape energy into particular form (or essence); the amount of mind power and energy involved is colossally different.

Merging one's mind with the Universal Mind is a necessary process for the performance of miracles. The *Art of Wisdom*, described in the previous chapter, is an excellent exercise for this

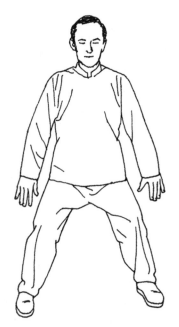

*Fig. 20.1 Big Universe*

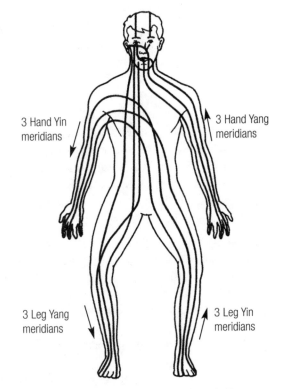

3 Hand Yin meridians

3 Hand Yang meridians

3 Leg Yang meridians

3 Leg Yin meridians

*Fig. 20.2 Hand and Leg Meridians (Partial)*

purpose. Another excellent one is the *Big Universe*, or *Macrocosmic Energy Flow*, whereby chi is circulated throughout all the twelve primary meridians (see Chapter 4).

### Achieving the Big Universe

The *Big Universe* is an advanced Chi Kung exercise, where training without a master's supervision is likely to cause serious internal injury. Hence, it is summarized here simply to satisfy your curiosity, not for self learning.

There are two versions, the *Gentle Big Universe*, where *Abdominal Breathing* is used, and the *Forceul Big Universe*, where chest breathing is used.

Stand in the *Cosmos Stance*. Start with a few rounds of *Small Universe Breathing*. With proper coordination of abdominal or chest breathing, let vital energy flow down the three *yin* meridians of the hand to the finger tips, then up the three *yang* meridians of the hand to the head. Next, let vital energy flow along the three *yang* meridians of the leg from the head through the body to the toes, then along the three *yin* meridians of the leg from the toes up through the body to the chest, where the flow continues into the three *yin* meridians of the hand.

In the second, or internal, stage, with proper breathing coordination, let vital energy flow along all the twelve primary meridians, emphasizing them individually and visualizing vital energy cleansing and nourishing the respective internal organs.

In the meditation stage, psychically see and feel vital energy flowing harmoniously through all the twelve primary meridian systems, including their branch meridians and internal organs. Then let the vital energy permeate every cell of the body, and expand outwardly so that the vital energy of the body merges with the cosmic energy of the universe, and let your mind be united with the Universal Mind.

# CHAPTER TWENTY ONE

## Chi Kung and Spiritual Fulfillment

"God speaks to the ears of every heart, but it is not every heart that hears Him;" nevertheless, he who seeks, finds—sooner or later— and to everyone is given the meeting he deserves.

Dr. Pierre Schmidt

### The Unity of Religions and Science

One of my most beautiful discoveries in the practice of Chi Kung is that, fundamentally, all great religions aim at the same goal. It has to be so, if there is only one Truth or Reality, although it can be interpreted differently and realized at different levels.

Outwardly, the world's great religions appear different, but if we go deeply into the teachings of their saints and greatest masters, we find not only that their ultimate aim is the same, but that their elemental approach is also similar. Interestingly, science is reaching similar conclusions too.

At the beginning of the twentieth century, Einstein's theory of relativity shook the world view of classical physics when he expounded that space and time are not absolute, but relative, and that mass and energy are interchangeable. Earlier, the result of Thomas Young's simple, but historic, experiment of passing sunlight through two vertical slits led scientists to ponder if photons had consciousness!

Max Planck discovered that energy is not emitted continuously, but in "packets" called quanta, which are particles. Louis de Broglie shocked his contemporaries when he proposed

that not only are waves particles, but particles are also waves; he was later proved correct, and this concept is now commonly known as Bohr's Principle of Complementarity. Heisenburg completed the shattering of the mechanistic view of the world with his Principle of Uncertainty, which states that we cannot be certain of both the position and the momentum of a particle at the same time, suggesting that there is no objective reality.

These and other exciting discoveries forced scientists to change their old, deterministic, mechanical view of the universe to one that is surprisingly similar to what has long been suggested by many mystics and spiritual teachers. Sir James Jeans, in his frequently quoted passage, says:

> The Universe begins to look more like a great thought than a great machine. Mind no longer appears as an accidental intruder into the world of matter; we are beginning to suspect that we ought rather to hail it as the creator and governor of the world of matter. [25]

### The Wonders of Mind and Consciousness

For millennia, man has wondered at his mind or consciousness and sought answers to questions about his origins and his destination.

The following quotation expresses his preoccupation with such wonders.

> A human being is part of the whole, called by us "Universe," a part limited in time and space. He experiences himself, his thoughts and feelings as something separated from the rest, a kind of optical delusion, of his consciousness. The delusion is a kind of prison for us, restricting us to our personal desires, and to affection for a few persons nearest to us. Our task must be to free ourselves from this prison by widening our circle of compassion to embrace all living creatures, and the whole of nature in its beauty.

Who do you think said these inspiring words? Not a mystic nor a spiritual teacher, as you may have thought, but one of the greatest scientists of all time—Albert Einstein. [26]

Chi Kung provides an effective means for man to find answers to his questions about mind and consciousness, and to gain a spiritual realization of his origins and destination. In fact, the supreme achievement of Chi Kung is spiritual fulfillment, irrespective of the religion the adept follows—or does not follow.

All the great religions of the world can be viewed from two levels: the popular, ritualistic level of the common people, and the higher, philosophical level of the religious masters. Most followers understand religion at the ritualistic plane, and are usually ignorant of the philosophical dimension. Because of historical, geographical, cultural, linguistic, intellectual and other factors, the world's religions are distinctly different at the ritualistic level. But when we study their philosophical level as shown in the works and teachings of their great teachers, we find that they are surprisingly similar.

We shall examine, in chronological order, the aims and methods of the world's great religions as taught by some of their greatest teachers, and we shall demonstrate these with quotations from the masters themselves.

## Hinduism - Uniting Atman with Brahman

At the ritualistic level, there are countless gods and goddesses in Hinduism; at the philosophical level, they are all manifestations of one Supreme Reality, known as Brahman.

> Before creation came into existence, Brahman existed as the Unmanifest. From the Unmanifest he created the manifest. From himself he brought forth himself. Hence he is known as the Self-Existent. [27]

In the *Bhagavad-Gita*, Brahman speaks through Sri Krishna:

> Men whose discrimination has been blunted by worldly desires establish this or that ritual or cult and resort to various deities, according to the impulses of their inborn natures. But it does not matter what deity a devotee chooses to worship. If he has faith, I make his faith unwavering. Endowed with the faith I give him, he worships that deity, and gets from it everything he prays for. In reality I alone am the giver. [28]

Brahman is manifested in every animate and inanimate being as Atman.

> I am the Atman that dwells in the heart of every mortal creature: I am the beginning, the lifespan, and the end of all. [29]

Devotees can reach Brahman in many ways, but the best approach is through meditation.

> The form of worship which consists in contemplating Brahman is superior to ritualistic worship with material offerings. [30]

## Yoga—Union with God

One way to reach God or Brahman is through yoga, which means union with God. Although it is extensively used by Hindus in their spiritual growth, yoga is actually non-religious, and people of different religions can practice and benefit from it.

There are many types of yoga, such as hatha yoga, bhakti yoga, mantra yoga, yantra yoga, and raja yoga. Raja yoga is regarded as the highest, and approaches union with God through meditation.

Patanjali, the father of yoga, prescribed eight phases, known as the eight limbs of yoga:

1.  *yama*—the abstinence from doing evil
2.  *niyama*—observance of purity, serenity, discipline, study, and devotion to God
3.  *asana*—static posture
4.  *pranayama*—breath control
5.  *pratyahara*—withdrawal of the senses
6.  *dharana*—concentration
7.  *dhyana*—meditation
8.  *samadhi*—enlightenment.[31]

The first five limbs deal with moral and mental preparation, while the last three concern mind development.

Mind development starts with concentration. Concentration leads to meditation, and meditation leads to enlightenment.

> The purpose of holding to one subject is the real key to concentration....When the mind is poised and well concentrated the supreme Self of man becomes visible....Intensity of concentration leads to meditation....It means feeling the presence of God within. The highest form of meditation is to fix the mind on the Real, the Unchangeable.[32]

Yogic philosophy distinguishes between mind and soul (Atman).

> Mind is a finer body within this gross body. The physical body is, as it were, only the outer crust of the mind .... Behind the mind is the Atman, the real Self of man. Body and mind are material; Atman is pure Spirit. Mind is not the Atman but distinct from the Atman.[33]

The ultimate aim of a Hindu, therefore, is to purify his spirit and free himself from illusion (*maya*) so that his Atman is united with Brahman.

### Taoism—the Way of Immortality

Traditionally, Lao Tzu, who lived in the sixth century BC, is regarded as the founder of Taoism. However, many Western scholars, after a few years' study of Chinese texts, insist that Taoism only materialized about 300 years after Lao Tzu, whereas the people who have actually been practicing it for centuries say that it originated at the time of Huang Ti, the Yellow Emperor, about the twenty-second century BC.

At its philosophical level, Taoism is surprisingly similar to Hinduism, although there is no record of any significant mutual influence. While the ritualistic Taoism of the common people deals with countless gods and goddesses, the higher philosophical Taoism teaches the attainment of immortality by merging with Tao. What is Tao? Lao Tzu said:

> Everything comes from That which cannot be named nor described because it is beyond man's comprehension; but for convenience it is called Tao.[34]

Regarding Taoist cosmology, Lao Tzu explained:

> Tao creates one. One creates two. Two creates three. Three creates everything in the universe.[35]

The great wisdom of this saying becomes apparent when we realize that Tao means the Ultimate Reality, one means the cosmos, two means *yin* and *yang*, and three the positive, negative and neutral charges of energy.

Taoism shows a way to return to this Ultimate Reality, thus attaining immortality. How? A Chinese emperor asked his Taoist master, Wu Chong Xu, who replied:

> Morality is the first essential in the training for immortality. Then the trainee should meditate on the void. Once he is in meditation, he unites his mind with his breath, and eliminates all emotions and all cares, and just focuses on the void. The void means that which is before anything came into

being; it is the primordial of the extreme. Returning to the void means returning to the primordial origin, returning to the primordial nature.[36]

## The Unity of Man and the Cosmos

Basically, the Taoist method consists in developing the "three treasures of man:" essence (*jing*), energy (*chi*) and mind or soul (*shen*). The Taoist saint of the Ming Dynasty, Liu Hua Yang, explained:

> The secret of developing the pearl of elixir for achieving sainthood is none other than the function of *shen* and *chi*.[37]

This means that the secret to immortality is to meditate on our vital energy. The saint goes on to explain:

> The aim of sainthood training is to develop jing so that it forms into a shining pearl of energy. When this energy has been circulated through various energy points and returned to its energy field, it can be released as the immortal soul. Everybody wants to become a saint, but this method is a heavenly secret; hence very few people attain sainthood.[38]

Hence, the supreme aim of the Taoist is to attain immortality, and the fundamental method is meditation whereby the soul returns to the void, achieving the unity of man with the cosmos.

## Buddhism—the Way to Nirvana

The ultimate aim of Buddhism is the attainment of Nirvana, which is a state of enlightenment where the mind is released from the cycle of birth and rebirth. Many great Buddhist teachers have specifically mentioned that meditation is the only way to Nirvana. It is surprising that many Buddhists do not realize this important fact. Gautama Buddha himself achieved enlighten-

ment through meditation.

The teachings and practice of Buddhism are crystallized in the Noble Eightfold Path, which consists of:

1. Right Speech
2. Right Action
3. Right Livelihood
4. Right Views
5. Right Intention
6. Right Concentration
7. Right Effort
8. Right Mindfulness

The first five paths, which deal with moral living, are a preparation for the last three, which develop the mind for enlightenment. These last three paths are realized through meditation. In other words, a Buddhist may do a lot of good deeds, pray to the Buddha, even become a monk and enter a monastery, but unless he practices meditation he cannot attain Nirvana.

## Meditation—the Essential Path

The Venerable Dhammananada sums up the objectives of meditation succinctly:

> The immediate purpose of meditation is to train the mind and use it effectively and efficiently in our daily life. The ultimate aim of meditation is to seek release from the wheel of *Samsara*—the cycle of birth and death.[39]

Another great Buddhist teacher, the Venerable Paravahera Vajiranada Mahathera, emphasizes explicitly:

> In all time and at all places it [meditation] is the only means to the attainment of final deliverance, the eternal happiness taught by the Buddha as Nirvana.[40]

The same idea was expressed fifteen centuries

ago by the Venerable Bodhidharma when Emperor Liang Wu Ti, known as the Asoka of China because of the numerous meritorious deeds he did for his people, asked the master, "Sir, considering all the temples I have built, all the Buddhist texts I have translated from Sanskrit, all the good work I have done in the name of Buddhism, am I close to Nirvana?"

The master replied, "Your Majesty, I am sorry to say that you are still far, far away. All your meritorious deeds are a good foundation, but you have not actually started on the golden path of meditation to Nirvana."

Disappointed with the Emperor's anger at his statement of great truth and wisdom, Bodhidharma retreated to the Shaolin Monastery where he founded Chan (Zen) Buddhism, or the meditation school of Buddhism.

Zhi Yi, the first patriarch of Tiantai Buddhism, an important school of Chinese Buddhism, said:

> Avoid doing all forms of evil, practice all forms of goodness; ultimately let your heart [mind] return to its primordial, infinite void: that is the teachings of all Buddhas. There are many approaches to the infinite void, but the central, essential step is Zhi-Guan.[41]

*Zhi* refers to tranquility (*samatha*) meditation, and *Guan* to insight (*vipassana*) meditation. These are the two main categories of Buddhist meditation.

The main aim of Buddhism, like Taoism and Hinduism, is to see Reality as it is, free from illusion and impurities, thereby attaining liberation from the cycle of birth and rebirth; and the way is meditation.

### Christianity—the Kingdom of God

The main aim of Christianity is to return to the Kingdom of God. Although meditation is not specifically mentioned as an important means to

achieve this, it has been used by many Christians, especially those who have advanced deeply in religious practice, to reach God. The following quotations from two prominent Christian saints will make this clear. First, St. Francis Xavier:

> After this prayer I once found myself inundated with a vivid light; it seemed to me that a veil was lifted up from before my eyes of the spirit, and all the truths of human science, even those that I had not studied, became manifest to me by an infused knowledge. This state of intuition lasted for about twenty-four hours, and then, as if the veil had fallen again, I found myself as ignorant as before. At the same time, an interior voice said to me: "Such is human knowledge; of what use is it? It is I, it is My Love, that must be studied."

Secondly, St. Ignatius:

> This mind was suddenly filled with a new and strange illumination, so that in one moment, and without any sensible image or appearance, certain things pertaining to the mysteries of the faith, together with other truths of natural science, were revealed to him, and this so abundantly and so clearly, that he himself said that if all the spiritual light which his spirit had received from God up to the time when he was more than sixty years old could be collected into one, it seemed to him that all of this knowledge could not equal what was at that moment conveyed to his soul.[42]

How closely these experiences resemble those of the Buddhist, Taoist, Hindu and other mystics! All these ecstatic, spiritual experiences happened while the saints were in meditation.

### Christian Meditation

Dr. Johnson, a devout theologian and Christian minister who later studied under a living saint, points out that:

> All religions in all ages have had their own methods of silent meditation and of going inside and

developing inner experience....Devotees of every religion in the world have, to some extent, tapped the fountains of the inner life. This is true in Christian history as well as in all other religions.[43]

It is obvious that meditation does not necessarily mean sitting cross-legged with eyes closed and doing nothing. It can take any form. The crucial point is that the mind should become tranquil and be in contact with the Supreme Reality. Sincere prayer is a form of deep meditation.

St. Augustine described the techniques and philosophy of Christian meditation. His description clearly shows the similarity between the Christian and the Eastern mystics in their entry into altered awareness and union with the Supreme Being.

> Augustine advocated a long process of self-denial, self-conquest, and the practice of virtue as preparation for "the ascent to the contemplation of God." Only such ascetic self-discipline can bring about the readjustment of character prerequisite for entry into the higher stages of a spiritual life. Augustine is insistent that not until the monk has so become "cleansed and healed" can he begin the proper practice of what he calls "contemplation." Contemplation itself entails "recollection" and "introversion." Recollection is concentrating the mind, banishing all images, thoughts and sense perceptions. Having emptied the mind of all distractions, introversion can begin. Introversion concentrates the mind on its own deepest part in what is seen as the final step before the soul finds God.[44]

The ultimate aim of Christian meditation, as of Christianity itself, is to reach God, to return to His Kingdom for eternal life. Where is God's Kingdom? Jesus himself answered this question in the Bible.

> Some Pharisees asked Jesus when the Kingdom of God would come. His answer was, "The Kingdom of God does not come in such a way as to be seen. No one will say, "Look, here it is!" or, "There it is," because the Kingdom of God is within you."[45]

## *Islam—the Return to God*

Muslims believe that we are alive because of the breath of Allah or God, and the ultimate aim of Islam is for us to return to God.

Shaykh Hakim Moinuddin Chishti, an Islamic master, describes the aim of Islam:

> Every scripture and every prophet from the first have said the same thing: that we are created by a wise and loving Creator, and that the special purpose of our existence is to endeavor to work our way back to Him. Our objective in life is to regain union with God.[46]

How does a Muslim regain union with God? Dr. Mir Valiuddin, another prominent Islamic master, says that after purifying the self (*tadhkiya-i nafs*) and cleansing the heart (*tasfiya-i galb*), the next step, known as emptying the *sirr* (*takhliya-i sirr*), which is connecting the finite with the infinite, is achieved by *muragaba* or contemplation. Ultimately the adept achieves illumination of the Spirit (*tajliya-i Ruh*).

> *Muraqaba* is to fix firmly in the mind that God ever watches over you. *Muraqaba* operates at two levels: external and internal. External contemplation means "the turning away of the five emotional senses from the world and all its creatures; and disengaging from them both in society, and from vainglorious and meaningless thoughts when alone...."
>
> And internal contemplation is nothing but the "guarding of the heart" (*muraat al-galb*). "It is the preventing the heart from thinking of anything whatsoever, keeping it free from all vain thoughts, while sitting or reclining in public or in private, and disengaging from it cogitating on the past or the future. While engaged in contemplation if the thought of even prayer or worship comes, it should be negated at once, because this will bring contemplation from a higher to a lower level."[47]

Hence, meditation is very important in Islamic mysticism, that is Sufism.

## The Realization of God

Not only is the Islamic method strikingly similar to the methods used in other religions, so is the spiritual realization.

> *Tajliya-i-Ruh* or the "illumination of the Spirit" implies the filling of the human spirit with the effulgence of the Vision of God, and the fervor of His love….In all individual human souls the same Universal Spirit has manifested Itself according to the aptitudes of the individual essences….For the illumination of the spirit it is necessary that every relationship that the spirit has formed, after entering the body, with this world through sense of perception and knowledge, should be gradually severed, for it is their relations and attachments with this world that form a veil and keep the spirit remote from God. Anything to which the spirit is attached, and in whose love it is imprisoned, makes it its bondsman.[48]

The master also makes a very important point, which may apply to Christianity as much as to Islam, regarding the shallow understanding of the populace. Needless to say, "love" in the quotation below refers to love for God.

> According to the *Sharia*, *ittihad* or "oneness with God," if understood in the literal sense, is sheer unbelief and blasphemy….For those who look behind the veil, other than God does not exist. God is the only Being, and none exists besides Him….
>
> In the terminology of the Sufis, what is meant by *ittihad* is the state of the lover in which he is absorbed completely in the contemplation of his beloved, and in that state he does not behold anybody except his beloved (*halat-i-istighraq*). This is the highest reach of love's journey. Mansur al-Hallaj expressed this state in the following words: "I am He whom I love and He whom I love is I."[41]

## Spiritual Fulfillment in Chi Kung

This survey of the major religions shows that the methods of religious realization taught by their respective masters are similar to those found in advanced Chi Kung. Hence, Chi Kung can be very useful to mystics and spiritualists in their search for God or the Supreme Reality because not only can the methods of advanced Chi Kung serve their purpose, but the other aspects of Chi Kung can also provide them with the health and energy that their vigorous mental and spiritual disciplines demand.

The following exercise can help you to achieve spiritual fulfillment, irrespective of your religious belief. Sit cross-legged or assume any comfortable position. Go into deep meditation, using the one-pointed approach or the void approach described in Chapters 17 and 18, or any other method you find suitable. Then meditate on the cosmos, merging yourself into its infinite void and experiencing its infinite consciousness; or steadfastly focus on your chosen ideal, according to your religious or philosophical belief and see and feel the manifestation of His full glory.

The method is simple, but the path is long and exacting. However, if you persist, you will certainly arrive. And when you have arrived, you will have attained the greatest heights in Chi Kung, or in any human endeavor. What other effort is more meaningful and worthy than that of realizing our origins and destination, and actualizing the innate immortality in us? May your success contribute to the welfare and happiness of all humanity.

# NOTES

1. L. Watson, *Beyond Supernature*, p. 102
2. Xie Huan Zhang, *The Scientific Basis of Chi Kung*, pp. 168-72
3. Xu He Fan et al., "Elementary Studies of Chi Kung on Immunology", pp. 344-8
4. Xie Huan Zhang, *The Scientific Basis of Chi Kung*, p. 242
5. Bei Jia Te et al., "Application of Chi Kung to Promote Standards of Sport", p. 32
6. Wang Zhong Man et al., "Report of Chi Kung Therapy on Blockage of Swollen Lung Energy", pp. 170-6
7. Qin Zhen and Qu Zhi Ping, "Changes in Electro-encephalogram During Chi Kung Practice", pp. 201-8
8. D. Pearson and S. Shaw, *Life Extension*, pp. 15-156
9. Chen Yong Can, *Chinese Chi Kung for Nurturing Intellect*, p. 197
10. R. Restak, *The Brain*, pp. 343, 347
11. E. von Daniken, *According to the Evidence*, pp. 12-13
12. G.L. Playfair, *Medicine, Mind and Magic*, p. 23
13. For example, Watson says that critics planted magicians posing as psychics in a research group, with the express intention of deceiving the researchers at every opportunity. L. Watson, *Beyond Supernature*, p. 1
14. D. Goleman, *The Meditative Mind*, p. xvii
15. Lin Zhao Hui and Huo Xin Chang, "Research into the Effects of Chi on the Growth of Micro-organisms", pp. 51-3
16. Cheng Yi Shan, *Ancient Chinese Thinking on Qi*, p. 125
17. L. Watson, *Beyond Supernature*, p. 2.
18. Wu Xia Hua (ed.), *ESP Cases in China*, pp. 117-28
19. P. Yogananda, *Autobiography of a Yogi*, pp. 306-19
20. W. Anderson, *Open Secrets*, pp. 143-9
21. S. Ostrander and L. Schroeder, *Psychic Discoveries Behind the Iron Curtain*, pp. 41-57
22. D. Agee, *Edgar Cayce on ESP*, pp. 8-9
23. S. Ostrander and L. Schroeder, *Psychic Discoveries Behind the Iron Curtain*, pp. 46, 57
24. P. Yogananda, *Autobiography of a Yogi*, pp. 270-1
25. Sir James Jeans, *The Mysterious Universe*, Cambridge University Press, 1937
26. L. LeShan, *Clairvoyant Reality*, p. 142.
27. Swami Prabhavananda and F. Manchester (trans.), *The Upanishads*, p. 56.
28. Swami Prabhavananda and C. Isherwood (trans.), *Bhagavad-Gita*, p. 73
29. Ibid., p. 88
30. Ibid., p. 54
31. Swami Prabhavananda and C. Isherwood (trans.), *Patanjali Yoga Sutras*
32. Swami Paramananda, *Concentration and Meditation*, pp. 18-48
33. Swami Budhananda, *The Mind and Its Control*, p. 20
34. Xu jing et al. (ed.), *The Four Great Chi Kung Classics of China*, pp. 9-10
35. *Tao Te Ching*, Verse 42
36. Wu Chong Xu, *The Superior Combined Path of the Taoist and the Buddhist in Attaining Immortality*, pp. 13-15.
37. Liu Hua Yang, *The Principles of Meditation in the Attainment of Sainthood*, p. 20
38. Ibid., p. 20
39. K. Sri Dhammananada, *Meditation: The Only Way*, p. 33
40. P. V. Mahathera, *Buddhist Meditation in Theory and Practice*, preface
41. Bai Lian, *Introduction to Buddhist Meditation*, pp. 10-12
42. J. Johnson, *The Path of the Masters*, pp. 327-32
43. Ibid., p. 326
44. Ibid., pp. 57-8
45. Luke 17: 20
46. Shaykh H.M. Chishti, *The Book of Sufi Healing*, p. 23
47. M. Valiuddin, *Contemplative Disciplines in Sufism*, p. 97
48. Ibid., pp. 137, 143, 145
49. Ibid., pp. 159-60

# GLOSSARY

## A

**Abdominal Breathing:** The Chi Kung technique of breathing cosmic energy into, and storing it at the abdomen.

**Absorbing the Moon's Essence:** The Chi Kung technique of tapping the essence of the moon.

**Art of Lifting the Anus:** The Chi Kung technique of lifting and relaxing the anus.

**Art of Lightness:** A specialized kungfu skill for running fast over long distances and jumping great heights.

**Art of Retaining Gold:** The Taoist Chi Kung technique of refraining ejaculating so as to prolong sexual intercourse.

**Art of Returning to Spring:** The Taoist Chi Kung art of maintaining youthfulness.

**Art of a Thousand Steps:** The Shaolin art of running or performing vigorous movements without becoming breathless.

**Art of Vitality:** A type of Chi Kung that promotes vitality for health or sexual performance.

**Art of Wisdom:** A type of Buddhist Chi Kung that develops the mind for experiencing deep levels of reality.

## B

**Bagua:** Romanized Chinese spelling of *Pakua* (qv), or the Eight Trigrams.

**baihui:** An important energy point at the crown of the head.

**Beijing:** Romanized Chinese spelling for Peking, the capital of China.

**Big Universe:** The advanced Chi Kung technique of circulating *chi* throughout the twelve primary meridians.

**Buddhist Chi Kung:** One of the five major classifications of Chi Kung, which emphasizes meditation.

## C

**Carrying the Moon:** A Chi Kung pattern for strengthening the spine and promoting youthfulness.

*Causes of Diseases:* A colossal work on pathology and Chi Kung remedies.

**Chan:** Chinese word for the Sanskrit "dhyana," meaning "meditation." In Japanese it is known as Zen.

**Chan Buddhism (Zen Buddhism):** The school of Buddhism founded in the sixth century AD by Bodhidharma, which emphasizes meditation as the essential way to enlightenment.

**changgiang:** An important energy point situated at the tip of the backbone.

**Chanmizhong:** An esoteric school of Chi Kung derived from Chan Buddhism and Tibetan Tantrism.

**chenggi:** An energy point located at the lower rim of the eye.

**chi:** Chinese word for energy.

**Chi Kung:** A collective term for various arts that develop energy for health, martial arts, mental training and spiritual development.

**Chi Kung therapy:** The specific application of Chi Kung to cure illness, especially of other people.

*Classic of Elixir:* Regarded as the "king of al Taoist texts on immortality." Written by Wei Bo Yang in the second century.

**cleansing meridians:** Clearing energy blockage and facilitating energy flow in the body.

**Confucian Chi Kung:** One of the five major schools of Chi Kung, emphasizing mental development.

**Confucianism:** The embodiment of the teaching! and practice of Confucius and his followers. It stresses morality, education and good government.

**Copper Bell Stance:** A Chi Kung standing posture.

**Cosmos Palm:** A specialized kungfu force to develop internal power at the palms.

**Cosmos Stance:** Another name for the *Copper Bell Stance* (qv).

**cosmos-man unity:** A meditative state of mind when the adept experiences oneness with the cosmos.

**cuanzhu:** An energy point found at the inner arc of the eyebrow.

**cun xiang:** Thought retention, a visualization technique in meditation where a thought or at image is maintained in the mind.

# D

**dan tian:** Energy fields, especially the energy field situated about two inches below the navel.

**dao yin:** Literally, "lead and direct." It refers to a class of Chi Kung exercises that use physical movements to induce internal energy flow.

**distant chi transmission:** The sending of vital or cosmic energy by a master over a great distance to another person or persons.

**du meridian:** Governing meridian, which runs from the coccyx up the spine round the head to above the lips.

# E

**Eagle Claw:** A specialized kungfu force with a powerful grip.

**Eating Six Energies:** An ancient Chi Kung practice to tap cosmic energy. The ancient masters classified cosmic energy into six major types.

**Eight Trigrams:** A trigram is a metaphysical symbol of three lines, representing heaven, man and earth. The eight trigrams, which represent eight archetypes of primordial changes, are arranged in an octagonal pattern known as the *Pakua* (qv).

**emptiness:** A deep meditative state where the mind is emptied of illusions and sees reality as it is.

**empty sickness:** A figurative term referring to sickness due to functional defects or other insidious causes.

**energy fields:** Areas in our bodies where vital energy is focused and accumulated, similar to the Indian *chakras*.

**energy points:** Points on our body surface where the flow of vital energy inside our body can be reached from the outside.

**Entering Silence:** Meditative state of joyous tranquility.

**external force:** kungfu force that is easily visible, like a fast, powerful strike.

**external schools:** Schools of Chinese martial arts, mainly various types of Shaolin kungfu. *See also: internal schools.*

# F

**Five-Animal Play:** A Chi Kung exercise whereby the practitioner's movements resemble those of a tiger, deer, bear, monkey or bird.

**Five Elemental Processes:** A basic concept in Chinese philosophy. The five processes are those of metal, water, wood, fire and earth. They are frequently mistranslated as the five elements. The terms are symbolic and refer to the behavioral patterns, not the basic ingredients of the universe.

**Focus One:** A Chi Kung meditation technique focusing on one point or area inside the body.

**Fetus Breathing:** A breathing technique reminiscent of the fetus breathing in the mother's womb.

# G

**gen:** The name for one of the trigrams in the *Pakua* (Eight Trigrams). Its symbol is mountain.

**Golden Bell:** An advanced kungfu force whereby the adept can take attacking strikes without sustaining injury, as if he were protected by a gigantic golden bell.

**golden ponds:** Poetic name for the female genitals, from which the male sucks vaginal juices for his rejuvenation.

**Grand Ultimate:** Called "Taiji" in Chinese, the Grand Ultimate is another name for the Cosmos.

*Great Encyclopedia of Everlasting Happiness:* A gigantic collection of 22,817 volumes edited in the Ming Dynasty. However, much of it is now lost, and only about 700 volumes remain.

**gua (kua or trigram):** A metaphysical symbol consisting of three short horizontal lines which symbolize the interaction of heaven, earth and man. Eight sets of these symbols form the *Pakua* (qv).

# H

**Han Dynasty:** Period of Chinese history from 207 BC to AD 220 when the Chinese Empire reached its greatest extent, and its scientists were amongst the best in the world. Chinese today call themselves the sons of

Han, and what we refer to as the Chinese language is actually the Han language.

**hard Chi Kung:** Martial Chi Kung.

**Heavenly Drum:** The Chi Kung technique of gently hitting the back of the head with the fingers to stimulate energy flow.

**heavenly saints:** There are five levels of saints in Taoist philosophy: heavenly saints, godly saints, earth saints, human saints and spirit saints.

**Heel Breathing:** A popular Confucian Chi Kung technique of breathing cosmic energy down to the heels.

**huiyin:** An important energy point located just in front of the anus; the meeting point of the conceptual, governing and rushing meridians.

## I

*I Ching (Yi Jing):* Book of Change. Based on sixty-four trigrams, this famous book was widely used by ancient emperors and generals for divination. Scientists now marvel at the similarity of its principles to other, recently invented or discovered, wonders, like the computer and DNA.

**induced Chi flow:** A class of Chi Kung exercises whereby the practitioner moves about involuntarily because of energy flowing inside his body.

**inner-chamber disciples:** Disciples who are specially selected by the master for advanced training.

*Inner Classic of Bao Pu Zi:* An important ancient Taoist work written by Ge Hong.

*Inner Classic of Medicine (Nei Jing):* A very important book that crystallizes all the great medical wisdom of the Chinese from earliest times to the Han Dynasty.

**Inside Room Technique:** A branch of Taoist Chi Kung that aims to enhance sexual pleasures.

**inter-creativity:** Interaction of the *Five Elemental Processes* (qv) that results in certain processes generating others.

**inter-destructivity:** Interaction of the *Five Elemental Processes* (qv) that results in certain processes inhibiting others.

**internal force:** kungfu force that originates from within, as opposed to visible mechanical force.

**internal schools:** Schools of Chinese martial arts, principally *Taijiquan*, *Pakua* kungfu and *Hsing Yi* kungfu. *See also:* external schools.

**Iron Head:** A specialized Shaolin kungfu force whereby the practitioner's head becomes hard as iron, and is often used for attack.

**Iron Palm:** A specialized Shaolin kungfu force whereby the practitioner develops powerful palms for striking his opponent.

**Iron Shirt:** A specialized kungfu force whereby the practitioner is able to take strikes without sustaining injury, as if wearing an iron shirt.

## J

**jade juices:** Vaginal secretions, sucked in by the male during sexual intercourse for male rejuvenation.

**jing (channels):** Main meridians or pathways of energy flow inside our body.

**jing (essence):** The finest subatomic particles that constitute matter.

**jingming:** An energy point located at the inner corner of the eye.

## K

**kan:** The name for one of the trigrams of the *Pakua* (Eight Trigrams). Its symbol is water.

**Kungfu:** The popular western term for Chinese martial arts. Martial arts have been called by many different names in the past, such as *xiangpu*, *jiji* and *quanfa*. The current term is *wushu*, but the most widely used term throughout history is *wuyi*. Kungfu is spelled "gongfu" in romanized Chinese.

## L

**laogong:** The energy point located at the center of the palm.

**li (principle):** Principle. Confucian scholars believe that everything is made of *chi* (energy), and every action is controlled by *li*.

**li (trigram):** The name for one of the Eight Trigrams. Its symbol is fire.

**Lifting the Sky:** A very beneficial pattern found in many styles of Chi Kung.

**Long Breathing:** A breathing technique in Shaolin Wahnam Chi Kung whereby cosmic energy is channeled down to the tip of the backbone, then up along the back to the head.

**luo:** Branch meridians or collaterals.

# M

**mai:** The Chinese name for meridians,

**martial Chi Kung:** One of the five main classifications of Chi Kung, which emphasizes developing internal force.

**medical Chi Kung:** One of the five main classifications of Chi Kung, which emphasizes health and longevity.

**meditative Chi Kung state:** A state of mind in Chi Kung practice where the practitioner is at a subconscious level.

**meizhong:** An energy point located at the middle of the eyebrow.

**meridians:** Pathways of energy flow in the body.

# N

*Nei Jing (Nei Ching): Inner Classic of Medicine* (qv), an authoritative work on Chinese medical philosophy, herbal medicine, acupuncture, surgery, Chi Kung and psychiatry.

**nei guan:** Internal viewing, a meditation technique where the meditator views his internal body.

**nei jue:** Internal reflection, a meditation technique where the meditator experiences a thought or sensation internally.

**Nourishing the Kidneys:** A Chi Kung pattern that strengthens the kidneys and enhances sexual vitality.

# O

**One Finger Zen:** A typical Shaolin hand-form. The term also refers to an advanced Shaolin art of striking an opponent's energy points with a finger.

# P

**Pakua (Bagua) or Eight Trigrams:** The Chinese metaphysical symbol with eight trigrams arranged in an octagonal pattern. The names of the Eight Trigrams are *qian* (heaven), *kun* (earth), *zhen* (thunder), *gen* (mountain), *li* (fire), *kan* (water), *dui* (marsh), and *xun* (wind).

**Pakua kungfu:** One of the internal styles of Chinese martial arts.

*Peace Classic:* Written by Yu Ji in the Han Dynasty, the *Peace Classic* is the oldest Taoist text known today.

**Pre-natal Breathing:** *Abdominal Breathing*, the way a fetus breathes in the mother's womb.

*Precious Collections of the Great Song Heavenly Palace:* A colossal collection of more than 4500 volumes containing all significant Taoist texts before 1012.

**primary meridians:** The twelve meridians that flow through internal organs.

**Pushing Mountains:** A Chi Kung pattern that channels energy to the arms and hands.

# Q

**qi:** Romanized Chinese spelling of *chi* (qv).

**qigong:** Romanized Chinese spelling of Chi Kung (qv).

**qihai:** Sea of energy. It refers to the energy point about two inches below the naval.

**Qing Dynasty (Ching Dynasty):** Period of Chinese history from 1644 to 1911 when China was under the Manchus.

# R

*Realizing of Truth:* Regarded as one of the four greatest Chi Kung classics in history, written by Zhang Bo Duan.

**ren meridian:** Conceptual meridian, which runs from below the lips down the front part of the body to the anus.

# S

**sea of yang energy:** *Du* or governing meridian (qv). The energy of all the six *yang* meridians of the hands and legs flows into the *du* meridian.

**sea of yin energy:** *Ren* or conceptual meridian (qv). The energy of all the six *yin* meridians of the hands and legs flows into the *ren* meridian.

**secondary meridians:** The eight meridians that do not flow into internal organs, but act as energy reservoirs.

*Secrets in the Clouds:* A very important collection of Taoist works in 120 volumes, known in Chinese as *Yun Ji Chi Qian.*

**Shaolin Chi Kung:** A collective term for styles of Chi Kung (qv) that originated or drew inspiration from the Shaolin Monastery.

**Shaolin kungfu:** The most widely practiced style of kungfu (qv), named after the Shaolin Monastery (qv), Shaolin kungfu branched out into many styles, like Lohan, Praying Mantis, Wing Choon and Choi-Li-Fatt kungfu.

**Shaolin Monastery:** Famous monastery in northern China from where Shaolin kungfu and Chan Buddhism (qv) originated. There was also another Shaolin Monastery in southern China from where Shaolin kungfu spread overseas.

**Shaolin Wahnam:** The school of Shaolin kungfu and Chi Kung founded by the author, and named after his two most influential masters, Lai Chin Wah and Ho Fatt Nam.

**Sinew Metamorphosis:** A set of Chi Kung exercises devised by Bodhidharma for internal and external strengthening.

**Six Sounds:** A Chi Kung technique using six different sounds—*xu, he, hu, si, chui* and *xi,* which affect the liver, heart, spleen, lungs, kidneys and triple warmer respectively—to cure illness and promote health.

**Six Wondrous Gateways:** A famous meditation technique consisting of six steps: count, follow, tranquil, watch, repeat, still. It progresses from *samatha* (tranquility) meditation to *vipassana* (insight) meditation.

**sizhukong:** An energy point located at the outer end of the eyebrow.

**Small Universe:** Circulation of vital energy flow round the body along the *ren* and *du* meridians (qv)

**solid sickness:** Figurative term referring to sickness caused by easily discernible agents, like a virus attack or a structural defect.

**Song Dynasty:** Period of Chinese history from 960 to 1279. Pronounced and spelt "Sung" in English.

**Standing Meditation:** A Chi Kung technique of practicing meditation while standing.

**stillness:** A state of deep meditation in which the mind remains joyously tranquil, and from which super-normal abilities may result.

**Submerged Breathing:** A breathing technique in Shaolin Wahnam Chi Kung where energy is circulated to the lower energy field at *huiyin* (qv).

## T

**Tai Chi Chuan:** The English spelling for *Taijiquan* (qv), a famous style of Chinese martial arts.

**Taijiquan:** The best-known style of internal kungfu, whose movements, during practice, are slow and graceful. Pronounced and spelt "Tai Chi Chuan" in English.

**Three Circle Stance:** A Chi Kung and kungfu stance for developing internal force.

**taiyang:** An important energy point at the temple.

**tan tian:** Energy fields. Although there are many energy fields in our body, *tan tian*, if unqualified, often refers to the middle energy field about two inches below the navel. Romanized Chinese: *dan tian*.

**Tang Dynasty:** Period of Chinese history from 618 to 906, when Chinese arts and culture attained their golden age. Many Chinese, especially overseas Chinese, refer to themselves as people of Tang, and the Chinese language as the Tang language.

**Tao (Dao):** Lao Tzu, the founder of Taoism (qv), said that that Something which we would probably call Supreme Truth or Ultimate Reality, can only be experienced directly, and thus cannot be accurately described by words, but for convenience it is called Tao.

**Tao Te Ching:** *Classic of the Virtuous Way,* this short concise masterpiece of Lao Tzu, written in symbolic language, is the Canon of Taoism.

**Taoism:** Taoism is traditionally said to have been founded by Lao Tzu and elaborated by Chuang Tzu. However, many Taoist masters said that the philosophy and practice of Taoism originated with Huang Ti, the Yellow Emperor, in the twenty-second century BC. The ultimate aim of Taoism is to be united with the cosmos.

**Taoist Chi Kung:** One of the five major classifications of Chi Kung, which emphasizes breath control and visualization.

**Taoist Collections:** Since the Han Dynasty there have been many collections of important Taoist texts. The *Ming Taoist Collection* consists of 5485 volumes.

**Technique of Changing Energy into Essence:** The Chi Kung technique of transforming vital energy into sexual vitality.

**Technique of Raising Yang:** The Chi Kung technique of promoting male sexual vitality.

**Tiantai Buddhism:** An important school of Chinese Buddhism founded by Zhi Yi in the sixth century at the Tiantai Mountain in central China.

**tongziliao:** An energy point located at the outer corner of the eye.

**Tortoise Breathing:** A Chi Kung breathing technique that imitates that of the tortoise and promotes longevity.

**Traveling Dragon:** A Chi Kung technique with graceful movements resembling those of a dragon.

## V

**vital energy:** Life force. The energy in our body that sustains and operates all our life functions.

**void:** A deep meditative state in which the mind is void of illusions and sees reality as it is. Also refers to the infinite cosmos.

## W

**wu xing:** The *Five Elemental Processes* (qv), often mistranslated as five elements.

## X

**Xingyi:** Romanized Chinese spelling of *Hsing Yi* (qv), one of the internal kungfu styles.

## Y

**Yi Jing:** Romanized Chinese spelling of *I Ching* (qv), the *Book of Change*.

**yifeng:** An energy point at the neck behind the ear lobe.

**yin-yang:** Chinese concept of the two opposing yet complementary aspects of everything in the universe.

**yingxiang:** An energy point at the base of the nose.

**yongquan:** An important energy point located at the sole of the foot.

## Z

**Zhou Dynasty:** Longest dynasty in Chinese history, 1030-480 B.C., when China experienced her classical age. Often spelt "Chou" in English.

# USEFUL ADDRESSES

**Malayisa**

Grandmaster Wong Kiew Kit
Shaolin Wahnam Institute
81 Taman Intan B/5,
08000 Sungai Petani, Kedah, Malaysia
Tel: 60-4-422-2353
Fax: 60-4-422-7812
Email: shaolin@pd.jaring.my
Website: www.shaolin.org

Master Ng Kowi Beng,
20, Lorong Murni 33,
Taman Desa Murni Sungai Dua,
13800 Butterworth, Pulau Pinang, Malaysia
Tel: 60-4-356-3069
Fax: 60-4-484-4617
Email: kowibeng@tm.net.my

Master Cheong Huat Seng,
22 Taman Mutiara,
08000 Sungai Petani, Kedah, Malaysia
Tel: 60-4-421-0634

Master Goh Kok Hin,
86 Jalan Sungai Emas,
08500 Kota Kuala Muda, kedah, Malaysia
Tel: 60-4-437-4301

Master Chim Chin Sin,
42 Taman Permai,
08100 Bedong, Kedah, Malaysia
Tel: 60-4-458-1729
Mobile: 60-12-522-6297

Master Morgan A/L Govindasamy,
3086 Lorong 21, Taman Ria,
08000 Sungai Petani, Kedah, Malaysia
Tel: 60-4-441-4198

Master Yong Peng Wah,
Shaolin Wahnam Chi Kung and Kung Fu
181 Taman Kota Jaya,
34700 Simpang, Taiping,
Perak, Malaysia
Tel: 60-5-847-1431

Shaolin Wahnam Sabah
Dr. Damian Kissey
Sabah, Malaysia
Tel: 60-88-729-260
Fax: 60-88-729-548
Mobile: 60-13-852-0533
Email: drsanmat@tm.net.my
Website: www.shaolinwahnamsabah.com

**USA**

Master Anthony Korahais
Website: www.zenergyarts.com

Mr. Eugene Siterman
299 Carroll St
Brooklyn, NY 11231,USA
Email: eugene@cosmospublishing.com

**Canada**

Dr. Kay Lie
Toronto, Ontario
Email: kayl@interlog.com

Master Jean Lie
Toronto, Ontario
Tel: 1-416-979-0238
Email: kayl@interlog.com

Master Emiko Hsuen
67 Churchill Avenue
North York, ON
M2N 1Y8, Canada
Tel: 1-416-250-1812
Email: shaolin@shaolinwahnam.ca
Website: www.shaolinwahnam.ca

Master Anton Skafar
Shaolin Wahnam Institute Kitchener
13 Hermie Pl.
Kitchener, ON
N2H 4X9, Canada
Tel: 1-519-576-5780
Email: skafar@hotmail.com

## Austria

Shaolin Wahnam Qigong
Website: www.shaolinqigong.at

## Australia

Master Jeffrey Segal
Shaolin Wahnam Australia
Email: segaljeffrey@hotmail.com

## Costa Rica

Master Roberto Lamberti
Shaolin Wahnam Center in Costa Rica
Website: www.shaolin-wahnam-center.org

## England

Master Marcus Santer
Shaolin Wahnam UK
48 Brook Street
Dawlish, Devon, EX7 0RP England
Tel: 44-16-26-86-2756
Email : marcus@wahnam.com
Website : www.artofchikung.com

## Finland

Shaolin Wahnam Finland
Email: shaolinchikung@kolumbus.fi
Website: www.kolumbus.fi/shaolinchikung

## Germany

Grandmaster Kai Uwe Jettkandt
Shaolin Wahnam Deutschland
Munchener Strafe 12
60329 Frankfurt/Main
Germany
Tel: 49-69-9043-1954
Email: info@shaolin-wahnam.de
Website: www.shaolin-wahnam.de

## Italy

Master Roberto Lamberti
Hotel Punta Est Via Aurelia,1
17024 Finale Ligure (SV), Italy
Tel: 39-019-600-611
Mobile: 39-339-358-0663
Email: robertolamberti@liberto.it

## Holland

Dr. Oetti Kwee Liang Hoo
Tel: 31-10-531-6416

## Ireland

Master Joan Browne
Shaolin Wahnam Ireland
Mullin, Cordal
Castleisland, County Kerry
Ireland
Tel: 353-66-714-7545
Mob: 353-87-121-2249
Email: wahnam@eircom.net
Website: www.shaolinwahnamireland.com

**Portugal**

Dr. Riccardo Salvatore
Shaolin Wahnam Chi Kung
Praca Afranio Peixoto 2, 1°dto
1000-009 Lisboa, Portugal
Tel; 351-218-478-713
Fax: 351-218-421-174
Email: chikung.shaolin.wahnam@clix.pt
Website: www.shaolin-wahnam.planetaclix.pt

**Scotland**

Master Darryl Collett
Shaolin Wahnam Scotland
5/4 Saughton Mains Terrace
Edinburgh, Scotland
EH11 3NX, United Kingdom
Tel: 44-790-454-7538
Email: Scotland@ShaolinWahnam.co.uk

**South Africa**

Shaolin Wahnam Institute South Africa
Webiste: www.shaolin-wahnam.co.za

**Spain**

Master Jorge Leon Garcia
Shaolin Wahnam Barcelona
C/ Jaume Fabre, 2, 1°-6ª
08019 Barcelona
Spain
Tel: 34-669-871-141
Email: jleon@canneteja.com

Master Daniel Perez
Shaolin Wahnam Spain
Castillejos 433 2° 1ª
Barcelona
Spain
Tel: 34-650-389-120
Email: danielperez@net.zzn.com

Master Adalia Iglesias
Shaolin Wahnam Chi Kung
C/ Cometa, n° 3, atico
08002 Barcelona, Spain
Tel: 34-933-104-956
Mobile: 34-654-155-864
Email: chikung@xenoid.com
Website: www.xenoid.com/chikung

Master Laura Fernandez Garrido
Shaolin Wahnam Madrid
C/ Rafael Herrera, 3-1°C
28036 Madrid, Spain
Tel: 34-914-038-002
E-mail : laura.ferga@tiscali.es
Website : wahnammadrid.org

Master Javier Galve
Shaolin Wahnam Madrid
C/ Villamanin, 19, 5°-2
28011 Madrid, Spain
Tel: 34-656-669-790
Email: javier@wahnammadrid.org
Website: wahnammadrid.org

Dr Inaki Rivero Urdiain
Aguirre Miramon, 6-4° dch.
20002 San Sebastian, Spain
Tel: 34-943-360-213
Email: psicosalud2002@hotmail.com
Website: www.euskalnet.net/psicosalud

Master Douglas Wiesenthal
C/ Almirante Cadarso 26, P-14
46005 Valenica, Spain
Email: dwiesenthal@yahoo.com

**Switzerland**

Master Andrew Barnett
Shaolin Wahnam Switzerland
Landstrasse 118
7250 Klosters, Switzerland
Tel: 41-81-420-2250
Email: wahnamGR@bluewin.ch
Website: www.shaolin-wahnam.ch

# BIBLIOGRAPHY

I have referred to 196 books in English and 227 books in Chinese in the writing of this book, but because of space constraints, only the more important are listed here.

## Medicine and Health

Church, Dawson and Sherr, Alan, *The Heart of the Healer*, Signet Books, New York, 1987.

Fulder, Stephen, *Handbook of Complementary Medicine*, Hodder & Stoughton, Falmouth, 1989.

Huard, Pierre and Ming Wong, *Chinese Medicine*, translated by Bernard Fielding. Weidenfeld & Nicolson, London, 1968.

Jacka, Judy, *Frontiers of Natural Therapies*, Lotian Publishing Company, Melbourne, 1989.

Kenyon, Julian N., *Twenty-first Century medicine*, Thorsons Publishers, Wellingborough, 1986.

Palos, Stephan, *The Chinese Art of Healing*, Bantam Books, New York, 1972.

Pearson, Durk and Shaw, Sandy, *Life Extension: A Practical Scientific Approach*, National Library Company, Taipei, 1982.

Playfair, Guy Lyon, *Medicine, Mind and Magic*, Aquarian Press, Wellingborough, 1987.

Stanway, Andrew, *Alternative Medicine: A Guide to Natural Therapies*, Rigby, Adelaide, 1979.

## Science

Alfven, Hannes, *Worlds-Antiworlds: Antimatter in Cosmology*, translated by Rudy Feichtner, Freeman & Company, San Francisco, 1966.

Asimov, Isaac, *Asimov's New Guide to Science*, Penguin Books, London, 1987.

Capra, Fritjof, *The Tao of Physics*, Bantam Books, Toronto, 1984.

Harrison, Edward R., *Cosmology: The Science of the Universe*, Cambridge University Press, Cambridge, 1981.

Hawking, Stephen W., *A Brief History of Time*, Bantam Books, New York, 1989.

Koyre, Alexandre, *From the Closed World to the Infinite Universe*, Johns Hopkins University Press, Baltimore, 1970.

Morris, Richard, *The Nature of Reality*, McGraw Hill, New York, 1987.

Restak, Richard, *The Brain*, Bantam Books, Toronto, 1984.

Rousseau, Pierre, *The Limits of Science*, translation edited by John Newell, Scientific Book Club, London, 1967.

Zukav, Gary, *The Dancing Wu Li Masters: An Overview of the New Physics*, Bantam Books, New York, 1989.

## Chi Kung and Martial Arts

Bei Jia Te et al., "Application of Chi Kung to promote Standards of Sport," in *Chi Kung Magazine*, Vol. 3, No. 1. 1982 (in Chinese).

Chen Yong Can, *Chinese Chi Kung for Nurturing Intellect*, Jiangsu Science and Technology Publications, Jiangsu, 1989 (in Chinese).

Cheng Yi Shan, *Ancient Chinese Thinking on Qi*, Hupei People's Publications, Hupei, 1986 (in Chinese).

Crompton, Paul, *The Elements of Tai Chi*, Element Books, Shaftesbury, 1990.

Klein, Bob, *Movements of Magic: The Spirit of T'ai-Chi-Ch'uan*, Aquarian Press, Wellingborough, 1984.

Lin Zhao Hui and Huo Xin Chang, "Research into the Effects of Qi on the Growth of Microorganisms," in *Chi Kung Magazine*, Vol. 2, 1988, (in Chinese).

Pike, Geoff *The Power of Ch'i*, Bay Books, London, undated.

Qin Zhen and Qu Zhi Ping, "Changes in Electro-encephalogram During Chi Kung Practice," in Tao Bing Fu and Yang Wei He (eds.), *Fine Collections of Chi Kung Therapeutic Techniques*, Book 1, People's Health Publishing House, Beijing, 1980 (in Chinese).

Wang Zhong Man et al., "Report of Chi Kung Therapy on Blockage of Swollen Lung Energy," in Tao Bing Fu and Yang Wei He (eds.), *Fine Collections of Chi Kung Therapeutic Techniques*, Book 1, People's Health Publishing House, Beijing, 1980 (in Chinese).

Xie Huan Zhang, *The Scientific Basis of Chi Kung*, University of Science and Technology Publishing House, Beijing, 1988 (in Chinese).

Xu He Fen et al., "Elementary Studies of Chi Kung on Immunology," in Hu Hai Chang et al. (eds.) *Collection of Chi Kung Scientific Reports*, University of Science and Technology Publishing House, Beijing, 1989 (in Chinese).

Xu Jing et al., *The Four Great Chi Kung Classics of China*, Jijiang Classical Book Publishers, Jijiang, 1988 (in Chinese).

Yang Jwing-Ming, *The Root of Chinese Chi Kung*, Yang's Martial Arts Association, Jamaica Plain, 1989.

## ESP, Psi and Metaphysics

Agee, Doris, *Edgar Cayce on ESP*, Warner Books, New York, 1988.

Butler, W.E., *How to Read the Aura, Practice Psychometry, Telepathy and Clairvoyance*, Destiny Books, Rochester, 1987.

Cayce, Edgar, *Edgar Cayce: Modern Prophet*, Bonanza Books, New York, 1990.

Crawford, Quantz, *Methods of Psychic Development*, Samuel Weiser, York Beach, 1988.

Gawain, Shakti, *Creative Visualization*, Bantam Books, New York, 1985.

Inglis, Brian, *Science and Parascience*, Hodder & Stoughton, London, 1984.

—*Trance: A Natural History of Altered States of Mind*, Paladin Books, London, 1990.

LeShan, Lawrence, *Clairvoyant Reality*, Turnstone Press, Wellingborough, 1982.

MacLaine, Shirley, *Going Within*, Bantam Books, New York, 1990.

Mishlove, Jeffrey, *Psi Development Systems*, Ballantine Books, New York, 1988.

Moody, Raymond A. Jr., *Life After Life*, Bantam Books, Toronto, 1988.

Muldoon, Sylvan and Carrington, Hereward, *The Projection of the Astral Body*, Rider, London, 1989.

Murphy, Joseph, *The Power of Your Subconscious Mind*, Bantam Books, Toronto, 1985.

Ostrander, Sheila and Schroeder, Lynn, *Psychic Discoveries Behind the Iron Curtain*, Prentice Hall, Eaglewood Cliffs, 1970.

Radnor, Alan, *Paranormal or Normal*, Lennard Publishing, London, 1989.

Robert, Jane, *How To Develop your ESP Powers*, Rider, London, 1988.

Rogo, D. Scott, *Leaving the Body*, Prentice Hall, New York, 1983.

—*Our Psychic Potentials*, Prentice Hall, New York, 1984.

Sherman, Harold, *How to Make ESP Work for You*, Fawcett Crest, New York, 1988.

—*Your Mysterious Powers of ESP*, Signet Books, New York, 1988.

Stone, Robert B., *The Power of Miracle Metaphysics*, Parker Publishing Company, New York, 2987.

Weed, Joseph J., *How You Can Predict the Future*, Thomas & Co., Wellingborough, 1978.

—*Wisdom of the Mystic Masters*, Parker Publishing Company, New York, 1988.

Wilson, Ian, *The After Death Experience*, Gorgi Books, London, 1989.

Wu Xiao Hua (ed.), *ESP Cases in China*, Wan Feng Publications, Hong Kong, 1987 (in Chinese).

## Meditation

Goleman, Daniel, *The Meditative Mind: The Varieties of Meditative Experience*, Jeremy Tarcher, Los Angeles, 1988.

LeShan, Lawrence, *How to Meditate*, Bantam Books, Toronto, 1988.

Liu Hua Yang, *The Principles of Meditation in the Attainment of Sainthood*, edited by Lian Yang, the Recluse, Sunny Books, Taipei, 1988 (in Chinese).

Mahesh Yogi, Maharishi, *The Science of Being and Art of Living: Transcendental Meditation,* Signet Books, New York, 1988.

Norvell, *The Miracle Power of Transcendental Meditation,* Parker Publishing Company, New York, 1988.

Silva, Jose and Miele, Philip, *The Silva Mind Control Method,* Granada Publishing, London, 1980.

## The Occult

Drury, Nevill, *The Path of the Chameleon,* Neville Spearman, Jersey, 1973.

Eliade, Mircea, Shamanism: *Archaic Techniques of Ecstasy,* translated by Willard R. Trask, Arkana, London, 1989.

Green, Marian, *The Gentle Arts of Aquarian Magic,* Aquarian Press, Wellingborough, 1987.

Leek, Sybil, *The Complete Art of Witchcraft,* Signet Books, New York, 1973.

Ridall, Kathryn, *Channeling: How to Reach Out to Your Spirit Guides,* Bantam Books, Toronto, 1988.

Stevens, Jose and Stevens, Lena S., *Secrets of Shamanism,* Avon Books, New York, 1988.

Williston, Glenn and Johnstone, Judith, *Discovering Your Past Lives,* Aquarian Press, London, 1988.

## Buddhism

Anderson, Watt, *Open Secrets: A Western Guide to Tibetan Buddhism,* Viking Press, New York, 1979.

Bai Lian the Recluse, *Introduction to Buddhist Meditation,* New Age Publications, Taipei, Undated, (in Chinese).

Chen, Kenneth K.S., *Buddhism in China,* Princeton University Press, Princeton, 1964.

Dhammananda, K. Sri, *Meditation: The Only Way,* Buddhist Mission Society, Kuala Lumpur, 1987.

Gyatso, Tenzin, the Dalai Lama, *Opening the Eye of New Awareness,* translated by Donald S. Lopez Jr., Wisdom Publications, London, 1985.

Jayasuriya, Dr. W.F., *The Psychology and Philosophy of Buddhism,* Buddhist Missionary Society, Kuala Lumpur, 1988.

Mahathera, Venerable Paravahera Vajiranana, *Buddhist Meditation in Theory and Practice,* Buddhist Missionary Society, Kuala Lumpur, 1975.

Ranasinghe, C.P., *The Buddha's Explanation of the Universe,* Lanka Bauddha Mandalaya Fund, Colombo, 1957.

Thera, Narada, *Buddhism in a Nutshell,* Harry Omine, Washington, 1959.

—*A Manual of Abhidhamma: An Outline of Buddhist Philosophy,* Buddhist Missionary Society, Kuala Lumpur, 1979.

Vana, Bha, *Practical Buddhist Meditation for Beginners,* Syarikat Dharma, Kuala Lumpur, 1981.

## Taoism

Blofeld, John, *Taoism: The Quest for Immortality,* Unwin Paperbacks, London, 1979.

Giles, Herbert A., *Chuang Tzu—Mystic, Moralist, and Social Reformer,* Kelly & Walsh, Shanghai, 1926.

Kaltenmark, Max, *Lao Tzu and Taoism,* translated by Roger Greaves, Stamford University Press, Stamford, 1969.

Lin Yutang, *The Wisdom of Lao Tse,* Modern Library, New York, 1948.

Lao Tzu, *Tao Te Ching,* translated by D. C. Lau, Penguin Classics, Harmondsworth, 1972.

Palmer, Martin, *The Elements of Taoism,* Element Books, Shaftesbury, 1991.

Wu Chong Xu, *The Superior Combined Path of the Taoist and the Buddhist in Attaining Immortality,* edited by Lian Yang the Recluse, Sunny Books, Taipei, 1988, (in Chinese).

Yu-Lan Fung, *Chuang Tzu,* Paragon Books, New York, 1964.

## Yoga and Vedanta

Bahm, Archie J., *Yoga Sutras of Patanjali,* Arnold Heinemann Publishers, New Delhi, 1978.

McArthur, Tom, *Yoga and the Bhagavad-Gita,* Aquarian Press, Wellingborough, 1986.

McCartney, James, *Yoga: the Key to Life,* Jaico Publishing House, Bombay, 1970.

Nikhilananda, Swami, *Man in Search of Immortality,* George Allen & Unwin, London, 1968.

Prabhavananda, Swami and Isherwood, Christopher (trans.), *Bhagavad-Gita: the Song of God,* Mentor Books, New York, 1975.

—(ed.), *Patanjali Yoga Sutras,* Sri Ramakrishna Math, Madras, 1953.

Prabhavananda, Swami and Manchester, Frederick (trans.), *The Upanishads: Breath of the Eternal,* Mentor Books, New York, 1975.

Sivananda, Swami, *The Science of Pranayama,* Divine Life Society, Tehri-Garhwal, Himalayas, 1987.

Yogananda, Paramahansa, *Autobiography of a Yogi,* Jacio Publishing House, Bombay, 1985.

### Christianity

Dupre, Louis, *The Deeper Life: An Introduction to Christian Mysticism,* Crossroad Publishing Company, New York, 1981.

James, William, *The Varieties of Religious Experience,* Mentor Books, New York, 1958.

Neil, William, *The Message of the Bible,* Harper & Row, San Francisco, 1980.

### Islam

Chishti, Shaykh Hakim Moinuddin, *Sufi Healing,* Inner Traditions International, New York, 1989.

Shah, Idries, *The Way of the Sufi,* E.P. Dutton, New York, 1970.

Valiuddin, Mir, *Contemplative Disciplines in Sufism,* East-West Publications, London, 1980.

### General

Bharati, Agehannanda, *The Tantric Tradition,* Greenwood Press, Westport, Connecticut, 1965.

Budge, E.A. Wallis, *Egyptian Religion: Egyptian Ideas of the Future Life,* Arkana, London, 1987.

Campbell, Eileen and Brennan, J.H., *The Aquarian Guide to the New Age,* Aquarian Press, Wellingborough, 1990.

Davidson, John, *Subtle Energy,* C.W. Daniel Company, Saffron Walden, 1987.

Ellis, Normandi (trans.), *Awakening Osiris: The Egyptian Book of the Dead,* Phanes Press, Grand Rapids, 1988.

Fremantle, Francesca and Trungpa, Chogyam (trans.), *The Tibetan Book of the Dead: The Great Liberation Through Hearing in the Bardo,* Shambhala, Boston, 1987.

Gilchrist, Cherry, *The Elements of Alchemy,* Element Books, Shaftesbury, 1991.

Johnson, Julian, *The Path of the Masters,* Radha Soami Satsanng Beas, Punjab, 1985.

Price, John Randolph, *The Superbeings,* Fawcett Crest, New York, 1981.

Richelieu, Peter, *A Soul's Journey,* Aquarian Press, Wellingborough, 1989.

Von Daniken, Erich, *In Search of the Gods,* translated by Michael Heron, Avenel Books, New York, 1989.

—According to the Evidence, translated by Michael Heron, Book Club Associates, London, 1978.

Watson, Lyall, *Beyond Supernature: A New Natural History of the Supernatural,* Hodder & Stoughton, London, 1986.

# INDEX

MAKING
THE MOST OF YOUR
VITAL ENERGY

# THE ART OF
# CHI KUNG

By the same author

*Chi Kung for Health and Vitality*
*The Complete Book of Shaolin*
*The Complete Book of Chinese Medicine*
*Master Answer Series: Shaolin Arts*
*Sukhavati: Western Paradise*

To obtain a copy please visit www.cosmospublishing.com.

For Wong Kiew Kit's web site, please visit:
www.shaolin.org